Sick Health Centres
– and How to Make Them Better

Gerald Beales BA, PhD
Research Fellow, Department of Rheumatology,
University of Manchester
Formerly Research Fellow, Organizational Analysis Research Unit,
University of Bradford

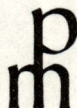

D1681095

PITMAN MEDICAL

First published 1978

Catalogue Number 21 0217 81

Pitman Medical Publishing Co Ltd
P O Box 7, Tunbridge Wells,
Kent, TN1 1XH, England

Associated Companies

UNITED KINGDOM
Pitman Publishing Ltd, London
Focal Press Ltd, London

CANADA
Copp Clark Ltd, Toronto

USA
Fearon Pitman Publishers Inc, California
Focal Press Inc, New York

AUSTRALIA
Pitman Publishing Pty Ltd, Carlton

NEW ZEALAND
Pitman Publishing NZ Ltd, Wellington

British Library Cataloguing in Publication Data

Beales, Gerald
    Sick health centres
    1. Medical centers – Great Britain
    I. Title
    362.1'2'0941   RA986
ISBN 0–272–79431–7

Set in 10 on 12pt. VIP Palatino
printed by offset-lithography and bound
in Great Britain at The Pitman Press, Bath

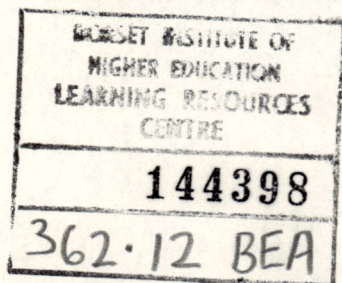

LONG LOAN

Contents

1 An Introduction   1
2 History   11
3 The Art and Soul of Planning   23
4 Drawing the Lines   47
5 Chiefs, and Chiefs and Indians   81
6 The Matter of Personalities   103
7 Managing It   121
8 And In Conclusion   137

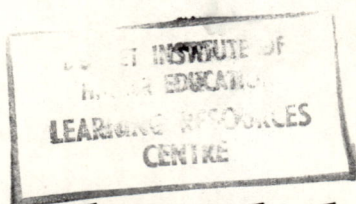

Acknowledgements

For commissioning and financing the research on which this book is based, the greatest thanks must go to the Department of Health and Social Security, and particularly to Dr T. Eimerl and Mr A. J. Forsdick. I am obviously indebted to all those with whom I worked on this research project in the Organizational Analysis Research Unit at Bradford for their inspiration (to the extent that I have been inspired) and for their companionship during this period. I must name Michael Wheeler, Dave Field and Professor David Hickson whose tolerance and encouragement made my time at Bradford so enjoyable and interesting. Judy Etheridge has made a particular study of the history of health centres, and she provided the material on which the second chapter of this book is based. She cannot be held responsible for any inadequacies of that chapter but I am indebted to her for her help and advice.

No research of this kind is possible without the co-operation and goodwill of all those people who are themselves the subjects of the research. Many people in many health centres have given myself and my colleagues the benefits of their time and their wisdom, and I am indeed deeply grateful to them for so doing. It is their good ideas, and their unfortunate mistakes, that fill the pages of this book. Obviously I cannot name them here, even if there were room to do so, and they have not been named elsewhere in the book. But they are there in disguise. Similarly, for the sake of anonymity, I have changed the details that do not matter when describing incidents from the health centres, but *every illustration presented in the following chapters is taken from very real life.*

Finally I must say thank you to Judith Hyde, Yvonne Prendergast and Doreen Ward for typing the manuscript, and to my wife Joan for being harassed by the children while I tried to think.

Preface

This book is based on research which was undertaken by members of the Organizational Analysis Research Unit, University of Bradford, from 1971 to 1976, under the direction of Professor D. J. Hickson. The research was financed by the Department of Health and Social Security, but the views expressed together with the recommendations made are not necessarily those of the DHSS or any other Government Department.

Preface

CHAPTER ONE

An Introduction

Health centres cost money. They cost a great deal of money, which is why they should be as good as they can be. They rarely are.

There will be some who disagree with this, who disagree because they see nothing wrong; nothing worth shouting about, anyway. Who will retort that health centres in general—in their experience—are really sound and fine establishments, much better than the tumbledown terraces that went before. So they may be. It all depends on your criteria.

Health centres have a habit of looking nice, being warm, and feeling comfortable. They are often welcomed so enthusiastically simply because they seem like palaces—in comparison with their sad and squalid predecessors. But beauty, as they say, does not go very deep. Pleasant surroundings are well worth having but they are not enough in themselves.

Apart from looking nice, the bigger centres look impressive too, and reassuring in an age of science and technology.

When one GP reflected on his brand-new, multi-storeyed, plastic paradise, his voice was broken and there were tears in his eyes. He said the health centre had given him new self-respect, and even the patients called him 'doctor' once again, instead of 'that old fool'. It was like it had been in the beginning, when he first came into practice, and before 'Your Life in Their Hands'. He said that as the years went by on Foundry Street, and as the little hut they called 'The Surgery' creaked louder in the wind, the patients had become increasingly sophisticated. They expected more than just a stethoscope and a sphyg'. Their idea of medicine was a heart transplant and sitting in his little wooden hut, he looked more and more like a man who did not know an electroencephalograph from a tea urn, and could not do a pre-frontal leucotomy to save his life. They took to telling him of medical research they had seen

1

reported on the 'telly', or what their daily 'paper had to say of some new drug, because they thought that if they did not, he would never know. The health centre changed all that. It had an air of hospital about it. Not too much, but just enough to indicate that everyone who worked inside it was both competent and cognisant: quite up-to-date despite advancing years. It did not seem to matter that he still had just his stethoscope and sphyg': that the minor ops, laboratory and radiology facilities that his younger colleagues had looked forward to, had somehow not appeared. None of that seemed to matter. Impressions are what count, and the impression that the health centre created was—impressive. So he was pleased. And, as he said, it may have done the patients some good too. He knew that faith counts for a lot, and such a reassuring place might be a powerful placebo. Some years ago a local wit had chalked upon the door of his old surgery 'Abandon hope all ye who enter here'. No-one would say that sort of thing about the health centre.

But even this is not enough. Health centres were supposed to do much more. They had a higher intention, and great things were expected of them in the way of changing and improving the delivery of primary health care. They were supposed to promote teamwork, and this is where the criticism lies. With very few exceptions, they have made a very bad job of it.

The idea was simple enough, and it seemed like common-sense, as many simple ideas do. Put everybody in one build-ing—doctors, nurses, health visitors, social workers and sec-retaries, dentists and chiropodists—and they are bound to work together. They will integrate and communicate, get to know each other, maybe even come to like each other. It seemed so obvious, but only because people have this curious capacity to underestimate their own complexity. People are not so easy to manipulate. The achievement of teamwork in health centres depends on a great many things. This book will deal with what research indicates are the more important of these. But first of all it is necessary to be clear just what is meant by teamwork, just what it is that one should be trying to achieve.

It is not enough to say that teamwork is a good thing, just as one might say that freedom is a good thing, or as the canine fraternity might say that a wet nose is a good thing. One has to be much more specific. On the face of it, it may appear sufficient

2

to express the hope that all who work within a health centre will achieve this state; that all who work within a health centre will consider themselves members of a single integrated team, regardless of how many people are involved, how many services or professions, how many practice groups, how many kinds of expertise. As far as it goes, it sounds a nice idea. But as it does not go quite far enough it is not only incomplete, it is positively dangerous. We shall soon see why.

It is necessary to make a distinction between 'the team' and 'teamwork'. In this context they mean quite different things, and comprise quite different sets of people. 'The team' really means 'the primary health care team'. This has been called the basic unit of community care*. It is the basic unit of any health centre. Its membership is limited, and is not dependent upon just who happens to be based in the same building. A primary health care team may comprise the total working population of a health centre; more frequently it will not. It will share the premises with other such teams, and with other workers not included in a primary health care team. The primary health care team is practice based. Normally it will involve a group of doctors, nurses, health visitor, perhaps a midwife, secretaries and receptionists. There are reasons, which will be discussed later†, why the social worker cannot realistically be described as a member of this team, however valuable a contribution she might be capable of making to it.

The desirability of such teams does not have to be argued. It is generally accepted. The health centre environment should foster them, encourage them, facilitate their integration, preserve their identity. This should be its primary concern. Its design and its whole style of operation should be determined by the requirements of the primary health care team or teams, which it houses. The secondary concern is important, but it *is* secondary. This is where 'teamwork' comes in.

In all but the smallest centres there will be more than one practice team, and a variety of individuals unattached to any team: health authority doctors, dentists, chiropodists, speech

---

* 'The Organisation of Group Practice' DHSS, 1971.
† See Chapter 5.

therapists, and others. They should not try to form themselves into a single, super-team. They should not be expected to. This is both undesirable and extremely unlikely to succeed. A team is a small and, in one sense at least, an intimate affair. Paradoxically, the bigger it gets, the more it changes into something less. It has to be small enough to know its patients, and for them to know it. But it is desirable that all who move into health centre premises should take advantage of the wider contacts that this move usually makes possible. As far as the primary health care team is concerned, goodness is not just a matter of internal relations. Introversion and isolation are dangerous, and they do not help the patient much. All but the smallest centres provide the opportunity to learn from others, to appreciate the skills of others and the contribution they can make, to liaise with them more effectively. This is what is meant by 'teamwork'. This is what should characterise the health centre as a whole.

Centres which house only a single team encourage isolation, and miss a lot of opportunities. But they also avoid a lot of the problems that larger centres suffer from. Large or small, most health centres fail to meet either of the aims set out above: they do not make for good teams, and they do not make for good teamwork.

Some might say that these two aims are incompatible—in practice, at least. That one either builds a centre which provides for the identity and integration of the practice team, and does without the wider relationships; or one so arranges things that practice team boundaries are broken down in the interests of 'extra-team' relations. But the evidence does not support this. It does not seem to be a matter of one or the other. Both have a habit of sharing the same fate. Either they both are met, or neither of them is. This is borne out by the fact that so many health centres fail so manifestly on both counts.

It is not all that difficult to see why, not if one understands what makes things happen in health centres.

People make things happen. They have this pleasing tendency to do what they want to do, despite all the constraints—physical and social—that seem to hang upon them. You cannot make them communicate more effectively with each other, you cannot make them work together more enthusiastically, you cannot make them like each other—not if they do not

4

want to. Human behaviour is a matter of inclination. Unfortunately it is not *just* a matter of inclination. There is always a price to be paid, and self-indulgence can be a very costly business. The benefits have always to be weighed against the costs. What this means is that practice teams and health centre teamwork will not come out of compulsion. They will happen if that is what the people want, and if the costs of operating these kinds of relationships do not exceed the anticipated benefits. The costs in this case are rarely monetary, of course, but they are real enough just the same: they are costs in time and in energy.

The health centre as a building, and health authority officers involved with the centre and its personnel, can do a great deal to reduce the costs of making and maintaining the sort of working relationships we want. Without going to a great deal of trouble, they can also make those costs so great that even the most fervent inclination falters and decides to take up golf instead. Too many practice teams, which worked effectively in their own little premises, are allowed to fall into decay when they move into a health centre simply because the layout of the building is so inconvenient that maintaining the team incurs excessive costs in time and energy.

As far as the inclination side of things is concerned, there is plenty of room for encouragement and persuasion. And here again, much depends upon the design of the building, as well as upon the actions of the people concerned with it. We all know how discouraging a wall can be, or how reassuring.

The aim, then, must be the *encouragement* of primary health care teams and overall health centre teamwork, and the *facilitation* rather than the hindering of such relationships. It is not necessary to choose between having teams and having teamwork. Both are possible. In fact, if an attempt is made to go for one at the expense of the other, neither is achieved. There would seem to be a contradiction between saying this and insisting that the primary health care team has to come first, with teamwork as a secondary goal. But in fact there is no contradiction at all.

The team is primary in terms of goals, not because it is most important to the welfare of the patient—although it may be; it is primary because good teamwork across the health centre as a whole can only come if the identity and the integration of the constituent teams is secure. The team has a lesser dependence upon teamwork, but there is still an element of reciprocity. A practice team that operates as a kind of social island is not a good team. It is not as good as it could be. The best teams are improved by a health centre environment that provides for closer working contact across team lines. This is why the smallest centres which were built for just a single team place limits on the heights the team can reach. Larger centres offer at least some opportunity to liaise more effectively with people whose work complements that of the team. But, more importantly, they also offer opportunity to observe closely other teams in action, and to learn from them.

Overall teamwork makes for better practice teams. But why is the development of health centre teamwork so initially *dependent* upon secure, identifiable primary health care teams?

When Dr Brown and his colleagues moved into a health centre only a short distance from their 'old' surgery, they did so without a great deal of trepidation. As far as things within their own practice were concerned, they did not expect a great deal to change. They knew, of course, that other people would be working in the building too, but it had not occurred to them that these others would interfere with, or intrude upon, their own working relationships. However, the sheer design of the health centre precluded the degree of independence and isolation which they wanted for themselves. For one thing, so many rooms and facilities had to be shared with other practices.

The time soon came when the members of these other practices were condemned as 'forever getting in the way'. Even the sound of their voices became irksome. Instead of living in harmony with everyone else in the centre, Dr Brown and colleagues developed a definite antagonism towards them. In many ways they went onto a war footing. The frontiers of the practice were stoutly defended: no-one was allowed onto territory which unequivocally 'belonged' to the Brown practice. No favours were granted to anyone outside the practice team. There was no question of working more closely with any 'outsider', or of communicating on any but the most formal and restricted of terms. But, in some respects at least, the team itself gained strength from this state of hostility.

Because they felt themselves to be under threat from outsiders, doctors, nurses, health visitors, and receptionists identified with each other even more strongly. Their solidarity increased, and, to the extent that they disliked everybody else, they seemed to like each other more. They were friendlier towards each other, more willing to help each other, and they had more respect for each other too. To a new and unprecedented extent, they appreciated what each could contribute to the welfare of the patients, and much better use was made of their various skills. So there was some kind of compensation, but the opportunities offered by the sharing of a health centre with other teams and services were wasted.

What occurred in this health centre was bad enough. But worse things can happen, and *have* happened.

Dr Smith and everyone in the practice team which (as far as he was concerned) he led, moved into their new health centre in a similar frame of mind to Dr Brown and Co. They, too, quickly discovered that things were not going to be as they had expected. They had to share reception and office areas with other practices; and their own rooms were often separated (and sometimes widely separated) by the rooms of comparative strangers.

These 'strangers' were no more responsible for this state of affairs than were the people of the Smith practice themselves. But human nature being what it is, they provided a convenient, immediate, focus for the frustration and annoyance which Smith and colleagues increasingly felt. Consequently, an atmosphere of disharmony, suspicion, and distrust began to pervade the health centre. But instead of defending the boundary of their practice team, the nurses, health visitors, and GPs who had previously worked quite well together retreated even further—to the doors of their own individual rooms.

Physical dispersal, and the intervening presence of outsiders having made communications within the practice team more difficult, these communications simply deteriorated. It was as if all had decided that their working relationships were not worth the extra effort needed to maintain them. Certainly, no-one made a deliberate effort to hold the team together, and consequently—it fell apart.

People have a tendency to fall out with people who stop them doing what they want to do. They also have a tendency to decide that they never wanted in the first place what circums-

7

tances make it difficult for them to have. What most doctors, nurses, health visitors, midwives, receptionists and secretaries want is a coherent and identifiable practice unit. This is fortunate, because the great majority of patients undoubtedly want this too. What they do not want to see is 'their' practice lose itself in a health centre 'soup'.

If the way in which the health centre is designed and operated facilitates and encourages the primary health care team, team members can happily develop wider relationships with no sense of threat or vulnerability. But if the health centre does not do these things, at best the team digs-in defensively, waging war—hot or cold—against everybody else. At worst, given time, there is no more team to defend. It is an error to assume that moving into health centre premises can at least do no harm: that if the move does not bring forth anticipated benefits, it will leave things as they were before. This is indeed an error. A badly designed, and badly operated centre can destroy relationships which were built up by great effort in separate practice premises over a period of years.

Health centres are not automatically or inevitably good for the practice team. Even the one-practice centre has its limitations: it encourages isolation and complacency. It encourages these things, but does not necessarily create them of course, for much depends upon the attitudes and determination of the people concerned. But even in such premises contact and liaison between the various team members can deteriorate, because many factors affect working relationships. Many factors can encourage or discourage, can hinder or facilitate.

Obviously, physical factors are important: the size of the centre, its internal layout. The production of a good design depends upon proper handling of the planning process. But the process of planning can do a great deal more than produce a well-designed centre. It can create a sense of unity amongst all those who will be working in the new premises before a brick is even laid. Much depends also upon the compatibility of the people who are placed under the one roof. Some people will never get on together in the same building, just as some doctors and nurses will never agree and never work together effectively. The problem of how to ensure compatibility amongst those within the practice team, and in the centre as a whole, has to be considered.

8

There are some ways in which a health centre is like a factory. There are many ways in which it is not. One of the latter is, there is no single boss; no overall authority. Different people are responsible to different people; some only to themselves. There is no recognised leader who can organise people into the kind of relationships desired. If there were, things would be so much easier. As there is not, it is necessary to look carefully at this question of authority, to see what sort of best can be made of it. Divided authority can easily make a divided health centre, and a divided team.

A related question is that of health centre management. Different health centres have adopted different solutions here. Some appear to have none at all. Management is not just a matter of changing light bulbs and ordering soap. The *process* of management, like the process of planning, can be a considerable integrative force. It *can* be.

But however easy things are made, however much encouragement is given, everything or nothing will ultimately happen according to what health centre people want and are prepared to make the effort for. However much is done, there are inevitably some who will not respond, because they feel that they have already gone quite far enough in the direction of the practice team, and who do not want the kind of wider contact that the health centre perhaps makes possible. This is sad, but unequivocably true. On the other hand, there are many more who would go further if the circumstances were propitious. But before going on to consider how to achieve this—how to make the circumstances propitious—it is appropriate to pause for an historical interlude.

CHAPTER TWO

History

Written with Judy Etheridge

Despite what Henry Ford apparently said, history is good for many things. It is often good for a laugh, and it is usually good for a lesson. And it can often help to explain why people behave as they do in the present. Our ideas, aspirations, and prejudices have frequently originated in times quite long ago, and we hang onto them despite their being inappropriate to the world as it is today.

What people today think of health centres, what they expect of them and what they are worried about, sometimes does not make much sense until it is realised what the health centre concept once meant. It did not always have the connotations it has now.

Having said that, it must be reported that the idea of a health centre originated—as did so many good ideas that still have to be implemented properly—in the early years of this century. Consequently, there cannot be anyone presently working in primary health care who could have been influenced by the very first debates, although many might look as if they could.

Right from the start the health centre was seen as a locus for teamwork aimed at providing comprehensive community care. The idea was to create truly *health* centres and not simply places for the treatment of existing illness. Maternity, child welfare and health education would therefore be given an important place. The general practitioner would be just one member of the team. This he might have resented, but at the time his worth in terms of community health was probably no greater than that of the midwife and perhaps less than that of someone whose concern was teaching the rudiments of infant welfare and the basic principles of hygiene. If *curing* disease was his primary concern, his contribution really could not be all that great, for the great development in therapeutics was yet to come. At the beginning

11

of this century the GP was still more or less in the position he had been in at the beginning of the previous one: he stood a good chance of being able to tell you precisely what was wrong with you, but very little chance at all of making you better.

What the doctor was really opposed to, however, was losing his independent status and accepting a salary from the state or local authority. This was what working in a health centre would have meant. It is easy to see a financial reason for this opposition, but the doctors themselves claimed a higher motive. They claimed that loss of their professional freedom would be to the detriment of the patients. In support of this they could point to the bitter experiences of the nineteenth century when the local boards had demonstrated time and again that they preferred a cheap practitioner to a good one. However competent and energetic the parish doctor might be, he knew that he would probably be dismissed the moment someone came along who was prepared to work for less. But the prospect of financial loss did help to strengthen their opposition. The Insurance Act of 1911 paid the doctors rather badly.

The doctor had to be quite an idealist to support the concept of health centres at this time and for some the First World War produced that idealism. Having witnessed the sufferings of the common men, they became committed to the provision of a public health service. Many doctors had worked for the state during the war and had found the experience to be not quite as bad as they had thought it might be. Socialism spread into the ranks of the medical profession. A body which called itself the State Medical Service Association (later to become the Socialist Medical Association) spearheaded a parliamentary campaign for a comprehensive public health scheme, with health centres and salaried service as essential elements of this. Reformers, such as the Webbs, envisaged treatment centres which would accommodate a range of health workers and which would be attached to hospitals—the GP would work in both, providing an important link between the different sectors of health care. But none of this came to anything. The great majority of medical practitioners remained firmly opposed to state control, and an administrative framework was set up which, in guaranteeing the independence of the GPs, firmly divided them from everyone else concerned with community health. Instead of

12

working together in shared premises, the doctor and the health visitor went into bitter competition with each other. The GP accused her of stealing his patients, and, as far as he was concerned, that was just about the worst crime of all.

When the Dawson Report was published a couple of years after the war, it gave greater substance to the health centre concept, but had no chance of being implemented. The GP was to be allowed to have his independence; he would continue to keep up his own surgery outside the health centre and inside the centre he would have his own private beds. Preventative and curative medicine would be provided for, and the doctor would lead the team. But the doctor was in no mood to line himself with the local authority side of things, even if his superiority over the nurse or midwife was to be conceded. Nor, for that matter, was the Medical Officer of Health necessarily willing to allow the GP any kind of say within his own domain.

Things had to wait for another injection of idealism. In other words, they had to wait for another war. The Beveridge Report adopted health centres with enthusiasm and so, for a time, did the British Medical Association. The BMA sent a questionnaire to its members. Despite the august origins of this document, only 50% bothered to reply, which must be some consolation to all those medical sociologists who find it practically impossible to get doctors to reply to their questionnaires.

Of those who did respond, a majority declared themselves to be in favour of health centres. Among doctors serving in the armed forces, 83% said that they wanted to return to a health centre when His Majesty no longer had need of them. The medical students were the most enthusiastic of all; 89% favoured health centres. Perhaps it seemed too good to be true; and it was. There was idealism all right, but the old doubts and suspicions remained. They wanted health centres only as long as this did not involve them becoming employees of the state, or coming under the direct control of the local authority. It was this fear and dislike of the local authority that forced Bevan to think in terms of executive councils and regional hospital boards for his new National Health Service. He knew that otherwise the doctors would not come in.

By the time the war was over, the idealism was already beginning to wane and the GPs were once again preoccupied with their professional freedom. The risks of losing independence were deemed to be too great and enthusiasm for the health centre was already declining by the time the National Health Service Act, with its famous Section 21, came into force. This section declared that

> 'It shall be the duty of every local authority to provide, equip and maintain to the satisfaction of the Minister premises which shall be called health centres'.

In practice, of course, the apparent compulsion did not materialise and probably a good thing too. It had become obvious during the committee stage of the Bill that nobody really had much idea about exactly what sort of places health centres should be. No-one had given much thought to how big they should be, how much they should cost, or how they should be designed or administered. In short, although many people were agreed that health centres were a good thing, they did not have a very clear image of what a health centre was, or ought to be. Nor could they be expected to have a very clear idea. There would have to be an amount of experimentation before construction began in earnest, and it would make no sense at all to begin a large scale building programme too quickly—not that a large scale building programme was on anyway, in the immediate post-war years. In 1948, the Government issued a circular instructing the local authorities to hold back on health centre construction, but it was probably unnecessary.

The BMA conducted another postal survey among its members in 1951, and demonstrated that human attitudes are not the most permanent things in the universe. Only 38% of GPs professed their support for health centres, which was quite a shift for the profession as a whole from the position of but a few years before. By 1959, when there were only twenty-three health centres in the whole of England, Scotland and Wales, the doctors were, if anything, even less enthusiastic about them.

Suspicion of the local authority was still a very important factor. The MoH was still seen to be governing his own domain in substantial isolation from the GPs, and generally showing little willingness to work with them on an equal basis. There were immediate fears that the patients might not approve of the change, that the doctor–patient relationship might suffer in the hospital-like atmosphere of a large centre, and that doctors consequently might lose patients to local colleagues who had remained in their own premises. But there was a longer-term fear too: a misgiving that health centres might be part of a plot to impose a salaried service upon GPs and to impose direct control by the local authority upon them. Instead of being seen as a desirable place in which doctors could join with others involved in community health care to provide a comprehensive service to the patients, health centres were condemned as impersonal buildings which would reduce the doctor to some sort of clinical automaton, destroy his status in the eyes of the patient, and perhaps ultimately put him in a bureaucratic straightjacket, stripping him completely of his professional freedom.

The trouble was that the GPs' status was already suffering a decline anyway. Not all the hospital doctors were doing well out of their alliance with the state, but the consultants at least were not faring all that badly, and specialisation gave them prestige within the profession which the general practitioner, as a generalist, could only envy but never hope to attain for himself. The public, too, were becoming more and more impressed by the great advances being made in hospital medicine, and the media did their best to make heroes out of the consultants. Technological hardware became synonymous with competence and expertise and the poor old GP, sat in his steadily decaying surgery, with no expensive machinery to surround himself with, cut an increasingly pathetic figure. He began to wonder if the patients really did want the guide and family friend he had always prided himself on being. Robots were all the rage just then, and perhaps his patients would be happier if he *were* converted into an automaton.

Perhaps they would have been happier, but it was not very practicable, so the GP had to think of something else instead. Knowing many consultants personally, he probably realised that most of them were not all that prepossessing as individuals, so when he asked himself what they had that he had not, the answer had to lie in their surroundings. The GP was, as like as not, all on his own. Some general practitioners were loath to give up single-handed practice, and some still are, but the benefits of joining—or creating—a group were becoming increasingly obvious. There were many practical advantages, but being a member of a group was often good for the doctor's prestige too. It made him seem rather more impressive. Apart from the GP partners, he might also have an imposing array of receptionists and other non-medical staff to serve him.

In 1963, the Gillie Report reiterated the advantages of group practice and introduced the notion of attachment of district nurses and health visitors to practices, replacing their existing geographical distribution which was not only inefficient but clearly divided them off from the GPs. Sadly the relationship between social workers on the one hand and GPs, nurses and health visitors on the other was largely neglected. However, the general practitioner could now have quite a team around him, and it was his surgery premises more than anything that still made him seem like one of the consultant's poorer relations. In the mid-sixties a high proportion of the slums in Britain appeared to have a doctor's brass plate insecurely screwed to their uncertain walls. There must have been many patients who looked upon a visit to their doctor in much the same way as their ancestors had contemplated admission to hospital. Sat upon mouldy furniture beside damp walls, listening to the clank of the water pipes, and watching the insects race each other across the rotten floorboards; crowded into a tiny room with so many other coughing, sneezing and poorly looking people, trying to remember who was there when he arrived and who had come after; not knowing how long it would be before his turn to see the doctor came, the patient must have wondered whether he was more likely to get better as a result of the visit or to contract something far worse.

In the towns and cities, the old residential areas were being abandoned by actual residents. Those who could not afford to buy something better at least had the prospect of a council house or flat to look forward to. The GPs, whose surgeries had once been so convenient, were now being left behind. The price of land and construction was rising fast, and few could afford to build their own new premises, or to adapt existing ones. It is not surprising, therefore, that at least some general practitioners began to look to 'the council' for salvation, just as the more hard-up of their patients had done.

The celebrated Doctors' Charter then made its contribution. It offered the GP reimbursement of rent should he choose not to own his own premises; in other words should he choose to become a tenant in a health centre built and owned by the local health authority. In strictly financial terms, the general practitioner might actually be better off by moving into a health centre and relieving his neck of the albatross of keeping-up his own ageing surgery. For some GPs the monetary argument might even be enough, although it was a bit like selling your soul to the devil. There was still the strong feeling that association with the health authority would ultimately do the doctor no good. Doctors who were having great difficulty in maintaining their existing premises might look at it in a slightly different way; the health centre was not seen as any kind of palace, only the last resort, rather like the workhouse of earlier days—to be considered only when you were truly destitute.

The consultants, of course, needed public money if they were to have the buildings and equipment they required and were capable of making use of. They had not got all they wanted, and probably they never would, but what they had got seemed exceedingly impressive when compared with what the average GP could muster. It would not have been so bad if the GPs had felt that they could not make use of better buildings and equipment if they had them, but the younger ones particularly were prone to the feeling that much of their skill and expertise was being wasted because they lacked the necessary tools. They were inevitably frustrated having spent several years training in procedures they were unlikely ever to be able to undertake in the poky little huts and crumbling houses they now found themselves incarcerated in. Furthermore, they may have been rather less suspicious of local authority and State than their seniors. They could be forgiven for thinking that if the Government in one form or another had provided the hospitals in which they had recently completed their training, there was no reason why it could not provide the means by which they might do a decent job as GPs. Some of the more imaginative and optimistic saw the health centre as the Big Rock Candy Mountain. Not only would it provide the sort of modern and attractive surroundings befitting their station, it would allow them to have a go at all kinds of things that *real* doctors did, and which they now had to send their patients to the hospital to have done. There would be X-ray and minor-ops facilities, and all kinds of diagnostic aids. Hopefully, there would be a complement of good-looking nurses too.

A combination of the GPs' declining status vis-a-vis the hospital consultant, the rising costs of buying and maintaining surgery premises, and the provision of the Doctor's Charter, led to a sharp rise in interest in health centres among doctors. In 1967 fourteen new health centres were opened, bringing the number built since the start of the National Health Service to forty-five. By the end of that year a further forty-five were in the process of construction and the plans had been approved for more than fifty more. The DHSS was delighted with the way things had started to go, because it was coming to realise that preventive medicine and primary care had not only been neglected in comparison with the big hospitals, they also offered—if properly developed—the prospect of a less costly National Health Service.

In 1969, fifty new health centres came into operation. By the following year, 8% of general practitioners were working in health centres and the proportion looked like it was going to carry on rising at an increasing rate. Another one hundred and fifty centres were either being built or about to be commenced. It was unfortunate that the programme had just gained impetus when the country ran out of money.

Sad as it may be, the inevitable cut-back in health centre construction has at least provided an opportunity to consider where mistakes were made in the past, and to try to ensure that they are not repeated in the future. If health centres are to go on attracting GPs to them when more prosperous times do return, they have to be much better than they have been. There are signs that the doctors are less enamoured of them now than they were a few years ago. To some extent this is because so many errors have been perpetrated in the planning, design and operation of existing health centres that even the most sensible enthusiasts have found it hard not to become discouraged. But partly it is because a fair percentage of doctors have retained inaccurate ideas about what health centres are and could become: those who expected far too much have inevitably been disappointed, and those who—at the opposite extreme—were prejudiced against them, have simply retained their prejudices.

There must be few general practitioners who can remember

the days when health centres were only mentioned in the same breath as salaried service and direct local authority control of all community medicine, but there are considerably more who have had their attitudes shaped by men and women who *could* remember those days. Doctors are trained and educated by older doctors and the young who are anxious to gain the acceptance of the already established are inevitably impressionable. They have a habit of adhering to the ideas and apprehensions of their teachers, unthinkingly, throughout their professional lives. And, in turn, they pass them on to the neophytes who eventually come under their charge. There are young GPs today who have been told—and have no reason to doubt—that the health centre is part of a plot to impose total governmental control upon them, and that the health authority is the enemy of their professional freedom. Old fears and convictions die very, very hard. Sometimes they look like proving to be immortal. But if they are to be changed, the first necessity is recognising that they do, in fact, exist. There are many ways in which the health authority can, if it wishes, demonstrate to the GP that it is anxious to work with him, and to help him, rather than to take him over. Quite a number of these ways will be mentioned in the chapters to come. Thoughtless action can, of course, reaffirm existing ideas, convince the doctor that his suspicions are well founded. Health authority personnel who are anxious to promote the primary health care team, and to encourage overall teamwork among professionals involved with community health, have to make a deliberate effort to convince any GP who is suspicious that his fears are no longer justified. On the other hand, administrators who themselves associate health centres with health authority control over the GPs, and who have relished the prospect for years, have to be shown that they are just as wrong as the suspicious doctors and have to be dissuaded from behaving as if they did indeed have the latter in their power. As for the poor disappointed soul who expects too much—or, rather, the wrong things—from the health centre, he has to be shown that although health centres may not be equipped along the lines of a self-respecting hospital, they are still worthy places with a great deal to offer. He has to be shown that in order to get back his long lost esteem he need not try to emulate the distinguished consultant. He can be honoured in his own right. Much of the medical profession already recognises this. In these days of antidepressants and anxiolytics, there is more need of a *family* doctor than ever there was, and more and more patients are demanding one. In a surprisingly short space of time the wheel has turned full circle. The patient finds it reassuring to know that there is available a hospital with technology to *analyse* him, but he hopes that he will never need it, and for most of his problems all that he wants is a doctor who *knows* him.

In order to deliver this kind of service, however, the GP cannot work alone. He can only do it as part of a team. And if the team really is a team, and all its members are closely integrated, the patient can be better off than he has ever been. But if doctor, nurse, health visitor, social worker are only loosely related, the unfortunate patient gets lost somewhere in among them and suffers all the more because he is convinced that nobody cares.

The health centre exists to allow the primary health care team to be as good as it can be, given the fact that it has to be made up of human beings. It also exists to help the team build up its contacts with others whose work relates to its own. But above all, the health centre has to be a place that convinces the patient that someone does indeed care about him, and that he has his very own clearly identifiable practice team at his disposal. If the health centre is not going to be equipped like a hospital it makes no sense at all for it to look reminiscent of one. The doctor mentioned in the Introduction did believe that his patients were impressed by an out-patients atmosphere, and that they thought more highly of him as a result. But they would probably have been much more impressed if the health centre had been an intimate and cosy sort of place, where they could feel they had a personal relationship with the doctor and everyone else in the practice team. Patients do not like feeling that they are merely numbers, or anonymous packages of symptoms crowded into warehouse waiting areas until somebody decides to dispatch them to their destination. The health centre has to be designed and operated with the patient–practice team relationship entirely in mind. This is the best way in which it can appeal to the doctor who is concerned about his status, or who is anxious to make the most of the training he has received.

General practitioners are not the only people who work in health centres, nor are they the only ones who matter, but they are the ones whose current thinking has been most often influenced by the historical development of the health centre concept. Everybody else is probably much less aware of history. But this does not mean that the health visitor, or the midwife, or the chiropodist, cannot adhere to an image of the health centre that is unrealistic one way or the other. They can resent being more or less compelled into health centre premises simply because they have an unnecessarily gloomy view of what such a move would involve; or they can be disappointed because when they made the move they had an exaggeratedly, unjustifiably, rosy view of what they would find. Whichever it is, their performance in the health centre will be impaired as a result.

Finding out what everyone expects from the centre, and trying to put them right when necessary, is an important step towards creating a successful health centre. A good way of going about this is allowing *all* who are connected with a project to get together in the early stages of the planning process to discuss just what the health centre means to each of them, and what they expect of it. But this would seem an obvious point at which to end this chapter and to begin the next.

CHAPTER THREE

The Art and Soul of Planning

Many people seem to make the mistake of assuming that health centre planning should be left entirely to experts. But this *is* a mistake. There are three very good reasons why everyone who will be working in the centre, as well as those who will be involved by virtue of the authority they exercise over others, should participate as fully and as directly as possible in the planning of the new premises. The first very good reason is that if they do not, the design may be incompatible with their preferred way of working. It may just be a matter of small faults and minor irritations, but if they are not put right the minor irritations can accumulate into a major torment. And, once the building is constructed, putting even small things right can often be expensive or impossible. The second, even better, reason is that involving everyone in the planning encourages them all to take a pride and interest in the centre once it is in operation; encourages an enthusiasm for the centre that may initially have been lukewarm or even non-existent. The third reason, and the best, is this: if everyone concerned works together in deciding just what sort of health centre they want, they are more likely to develop a sense of unity and a sense of shared purpose which can be an important first step towards the secondary aim of overall health centre teamwork.

The process of planning can therefore do a great deal to facilitate and encourage the right kind of working relationships. If it is not handled properly, it can impede things right at the start.

Some will argue that, in practice, it is impossible for everyone who expects to be involved with a health centre to participate in its planning. In all but the smallest centres, regular meetings to which all are invited may indeed be impossible. It may be possible—it is certainly desirable—to hold *occasional*, formal or informal, get-togethers of this kind, but these get-togethers would have their value in promoting social contact. They would be too large to make much contribution to the detailed discussion of health centre design. However, full and direct involvement of all is quite feasible, in the case of even the largest projected centre, if the planning process is organised into tiers, and if representatives truly represent.

Where only two, or perhaps three, practice teams are involved, the actual planning meetings could comprise several representatives from each team (a doctor, a receptionist, and a health visitor, midwife or nurse), in addition to health authority administrators, architects, nursing officers, and representatives of other services which might be based in the centre. Where six or seven practice groups are to be accommodated, this would make the meetings unworkably large, and each team would have to be satisfied with just a single representative. Whatever might be his merits or otherwise, this individual would undoubtedly be a GP. This can safely be taken for granted. In order to ensure that other occupations and professions in the primary health care team are not neglected, there would also have to be one receptionist, and one attached nurse, health visitor or midwife in the meetings which make the final decisions. At a lower tier, each practice team would have to meet as a team, and each professional and occupational group involved with the centre would also have its meetings. At these meetings, the representatives would be elected and briefed, and would feed back the decisions and discussions in which they had been involved.

Such a scheme can work well. But it can only work if the representatives do indeed represent: if they are, in fact, representative. No-one should consider himself or herself to be an automatic choice for this role. Representatives should be elected—not self-selected—however informally. At the same time, everyone should be represented by someone of his or her own kind. It is easy for the senior partner of a practice group to consider himself leader of 'his' team, and inevitably its representative (unless he cannot be bothered, and decides to delegate). It is equally easy for the senior nursing officer to assume herself to be the only representative that 'her' nurses need. To suggest that anyone else should be involved—as well as, rather than instead of—is probably to provoke an angry and affronted response. But, to be properly represented, the receptionist should have a receptionist to put her point of view; the nurse should have someone at her own level of the hierarchy. If this is provided for, they will feel that they have some importance themselves, and that they are expected to make an important contribution to the health centre. If not, they may assume that they are considered to be of too little consequence to be worth consulting; that, like children, everything has to be decided for them, on their behalf. And they will not find that very encouraging.

What has to be aimed at is true democracy, not its apology. And two of the bases of democracy are information and discussion. Everyone has to be kept informed, and given plenty of opportunity to discuss whatever has to be discussed. Representatives have not only to keep in touch with what their people want, they have also to ensure that everyone knows exactly what is going on, so that discussion can be soundly based and meaningful decisions reached. Communication is at the heart of the matter, and a great deal of effort must be put into this. Relying on 'the word getting around' is rarely good enough. Ensuring that everyone who should be involved *is* properly involved, requires deliberate organisation of the planning process—arranging regular meetings, electing representatives, producing and distributing detailed minutes and reports. But the time and energy so expended are very much worthwhile.

Desirable as it may be, democracy is not recommended for its own sake, but because it makes for better health centres. There are solid practical reasons why universal participation in planning should be aimed at.

'What a Place to put a Window'

A good architect knows his limitations. He knows that he cannot work in a vacuum. There is obviously a lot of satisfaction in producing a health centre that looks nice, but the visually most attractive craft can hardly be considered a success if it has difficulty staying above the surface of the waves. The real satisfaction lies in designing a health centre that actually does its job, and does it well. To achieve this, the architect needs help. He needs a lot of help from the people who will be working in the health centre, or who will be otherwise closely concerned with it. They are experts in the delivery of community health care, and their expertise must complement his own. Their wealth of practical experience must always be made available to the architect, and hopefully he will never be so stupid or arrogant as to ignore it.

In their early days, health centres were naturally dependent for their design on veritable virgins: architects who had never tried their hand at this sort of thing before. Now there is a corps of experienced men, but it should not be thought that because an architect has already proved himself, he can safely be left to get on with the job alone. Practice teams have their idiosyncrasies, and sometimes these require acknowledgement in the design. Usually it is just a matter of the layout of a room, or the positioning of a door, a window, or a sink: small stuff which can make all the difference, which can decide whether a practice team works as well as it did in its previous premises, or better, or worse. Therefore the architect has to know the people who will be concerned with the particular centre on which he is working. He has to get to know precisely what they want, and precisely what they would prefer to do without, otherwise mistakes are likely to be made. These mistakes may appear trivial, albeit irritating and irksome, and frequently they are, but once the structure is completed they can prove expensive or impossible to rectify all the same. Pillars, for example, are always popping up in the wrong place. There must be few health centres which have not got at least one pillar that gets in somebody's way. But when the architect is asked if it would not be possible to move it, if only by a few inches, his usual reply is that to do so now would result in a substantial lowering of the roof, accompanied by a marked compression of the walls, and produce a building with an altogether unimposing elevation.

Even those errors which can be put right at little cost and without risk, seem to be remedied only after quite considerable delay, and with appreciable disruption to the centre. This is bad enough if the errors are inevitable, but so much more annoying when one considers how easily most could be avoided altogether. Possibly most annoying are those errors which somebody is always promising to put right, but never seems to get around to:

There is a health centre in the North of England which houses two practice groups. For various reasons, the doctors in one of these groups took virtually no part in the planning of their new premises. When the centre was completed, they found that each practice had its own, virtually separate, reception area, but that these two areas were provided with only one door through which to communicate with the rest of the building. This door was located in a wall which clearly belonged to the reception area of the other practice. The doctors in the first practice did not get on particularly well with the doctors in the second practice, nor did they wish to be, at any time, in close proximity to the receptionists of the second practice. Given the fact that they were anxious to communicate directly with their own receptionists, this posed an interesting problem:

Problem: how to get Doctor C into Reception A without crossing Reception B and without crossing any lines or lifting him off the paper?

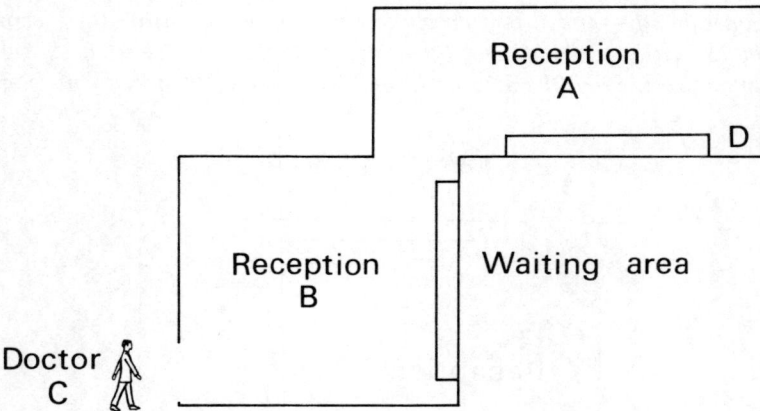

The answer is, of course, that there is no answer, unless you are prepared to cheat by rubbing out a line. This in effect, was what was decided. It was decided to ask for a second door to be provided at D. Surprisingly, this request was not greeted by mocking laughter and

condescending descriptions of the kind of catastrophe that would inevitably ensue should anything so radical be attempted. On the contrary, Doctor C and his colleagues were assured that such a door would indeed be provided. But nobody said when. In the following years, holes did occasionally develop elsewhere in the fabric of the building, but these were always unintentional, and none appeared at or around point D. Many letters were written; many telephone calls were made too. Somebody even reorganised the National Health Service. But nothing seemed to make any difference. Sometimes nothing does.

Most of those mistakes which are made and which could be avoided involve the design of reception and waiting areas. Receptionists are rarely invited to comment upon the layout of their own part of the health centre, or to say what they would like. Partly this is because reception is generally considered to be a peripheral activity of trivial importance, to which a great deal of thought need not be given. But lack of thought here can produce some hefty lumps to clog the smooth running of any health centre.

There used to be another health centre in the North of England. This centre housed three groups, and of the receptionists in these groups, none was asked to participate in the development of the design. Consequently—and it is probably fair to say consequently—they were landed with a shared reception area which came close to being unworkable. From the diagram it will be seen that the receptionists of

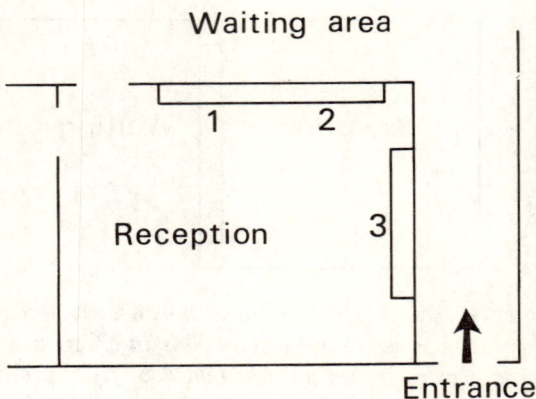

Waiting area

Reception

Entrance

28

practice 3 did not face directly onto the waiting area at all. They faced the entrance corridor. This meant that they were the first white coats espied on coming into the building, and therefore they had to deal with the casual callers, the new patients, and those numerous eccentrics who doggedly refuse to read signs. They also had a more substantial problem. The doctors with whom they worked had no system for calling-in patients directly. Instead, a light flashed in the reception area when a doctor was ready for his next patient, and the receptionist had to call the patient herself. Inevitably, these illuminations were not located in the vicinity of their own counter. Instead, they were to be found above the heads of receptionists 1 and 2. A congenital defect in which the left ear was replaced by a third eye would have been a genuine asset to these ladies. As none of them was so endowed, they suffered from chronically stiff-necks. And when the flashing light had been perceived, they had to clamber over stools, past filing cabinets and narrowly-separated rows of shelves holding the record cards, to thrust themselves between the shoulders of the other groups' receptionists and call for Mr Brown. Then they had to work their way back again.

Quite soon after it was opened, this health centre burned down.

Important as it is that the health centre design should take into account the current way of working of each practice team, health centres should not try to be reproductions of old surgeries, like museums of general practice with everything recreated down to the last detail and labelled in three languages. Health centres are supposed to be a force for change, and many people will want to come into such premises because they want to change things in some way. So the architect has to know how people will expect or hope to do things once they are in the centre; he has to allow for future developments. Great, indeed, is the dismay of a GP who hopes to do great things in the new health centre, and finds the building too inflexible to try anything new.

About a year after one health centre opened, most of the thirteen doctors who worked in it became interested in the possibility of changing over to A4 files for patients' records. In their innocence, they imagined that if they decided such a change were desirable, it could be accomplished fairly easily. However, as one of the receptionists pointed out, the

29

existing shelves for the records would not be suitable for the new ones. Larger shelves would have to be used, and as the shared reception cum records area was already extremely congested, this would create considerable difficulties. An arrangement would have to be made whereby only one receptionist moved at once, and even then the rows of shelves would have to be placed so close together that it would be impossible to actually get the records out.

This discouraged the doctors somewhat, but it did not discourage them too much. They believed that some way of overcoming the problem must exist. Consequently, they called upon the architect who had designed the building, and who was fortunately employed by the local authority. They told him what they had in mind, and he laughed. He reminded the doctors that the health centre was built on a sloping site. They retorted that they had not forgotten this, but could hardly see its relevance to their wish to change to larger files. Therefore, he explained:

Although entry to the GP floor of the building was on the level, that floor was not situated immediately above the ground. Underneath, in fact, was the health authority area of the health centre, which was also entered on the level at the opposite side of the building. This meant that the GP floor was supported by girders and pillars whose strength had been deliberately chosen on the basis of the weight it was calculated they would have to support. No-one had mentioned A4 files at the time of those calculations, and difficult as it might be for mere doctors to appreciate, the additional weight of many thousand larger files, plus the heavier shelving that would be required to contain them, would tax the strength of those girders and pillars very sorely.

Inevitably, someone asked if additional girders and more substantial pillars could not be inserted into the structure, with enlargement of the reception and records area at the same time. The architect said this might be possible. He also said that the work would involve the health centre being out of use for the best part of a year. Then he finished off what little opposition remained by doing a quick calculation of the cost on the back of his cigarette packet.

Sometimes requirements which the building will have to meet in the immediate or longer-term future can be discovered simply by talking to the people who intend to use it. There are bound to be other developments which no-one can anticipate, and the best design is undoubtedly a flexible design. Achieving flexibility without waste, without having empty rooms for a time (perhaps a long time), is certainly not easy, but it is considerably more difficult for an architect working alone than for one working in close collaboration with the people who are involved daily in the delivery of primary health care. Perhaps one should not worry too much about the odd empty room anyway. The short-term waste which it represents is nothing when compared to the waste represented by a building which fossilises future development of health care delivery in the community.

Sometimes the people who intend to work in a new health centre have to be reminded that their presence will not be permanent. Sometimes GPs have to be reminded that they will not live forever (and some of them, alas, for a good deal less). The idiosyncrasies which some may want taking into account may be too idiosyncratic, producing a building, or an area, or a room which no-one coming later would enjoy inhabiting. A health centre has to be personal to those who populate it in its early days, and yet be capable of being personal to younger people with new ideas who will replace them. It has to seem like their health centre too, not something out of the past that they have been landed with. Value for money means having a centre that is as effective and as useful at the end, as at the beginning, of its life. And a health centre should last a long time—God and the building contractor willing.

Therefore, it is not only a matter of those who will be working in the centre telling those who will be building it, and paying for it, what they want. The latter have to tell them what they can, and cannot, have. Many things which might be desirable in themselves turn out to be impossible on financial or constructional grounds. Fully involving everyone in the planning process ensures that they are fully aware of the reasons why they cannot have everything they want, or why the health centre has to have what from their point of view are imperfections. If people are aware of the constraints, they will usually accept them, and resolve to make the best of the compromise. They may not like having the window where it is, but at least they will recognise that there was nowhere else to put it. But if they do not participate in the planning, if they have not themselves been placed in the position of having to make decisions within all the constraints, it is easy for them to fall out with their new premises. To exaggerate its faults because they had nothing to do with creating them. To assume that something was left out because of bloody-mindedness on the part of the health authority, or added on the whim of the architect.

Ideally, when the doctors, nurses, health visitors, dentists, chiropodists, social workers, secretaries and receptionists turn up at the health centre on the first morning of its working life, they like it. They are much more likely to like it if they have played a full part in creating it. But even if they have been involved in its planning, there can still be some unpleasant surprises for them. They might still be heard to say 'did I agree to that?' Involving people in decision-making is not enough in itself. It is essential to make sure that all are clear exactly what it is that they are agreeing to. Deliberately or not, it is easy for the architect to blind everyone with his own brand of science: to blithely reassure that it 'may look a bit odd on the plan, but you'll like it when it's built'. And it is easy for everyone else to assume that he is probably right. After all, they know that they cannot trust their own judgement. They are not competent. Most GPs are about as good at interpreting blueprints as most architects are at interpreting heart sounds. When a health centre was being considered for a certain Lancashire town, the receptionists were privileged in being allowed to see the plans before a brick was laid. They spent half an hour perusing those plans, and still could not find the door into their own reception area. They were not dismayed, however. They took it for granted that there must be one. And fortunately there was. But it was not where they wanted it.

In the case of one of the largest health centres in this country, the GPs concerned were very much involved with the project right from the start. They had had their own, very clear, ideas on the layout of the building, and they had worked closely with an architect who was both competent and co-operative. All should have been well. But before the building was fitted out internally, the GPs paid a visit to it, and what they saw resulted in some of them threatening to withdraw altogether. One of the few aspects of the design which they had not asked about was the arrangement of the roof, or, to be more precise, the amount of light that would pass through it. They had taken it for granted that internal rooms, which obviously could not have windows, would receive natural light from above. They were horrified to find that most of them did not, and would be totally dependent on artificial light. The architect's insistence that it was not, in fact, an easy matter at this stage to knock a few holes in the roof, did nothing to placate them. And it required a great deal of tact and persuasion on the part of the then MoH to maintain the doctors' commitment to the centre.

The architect must go to great pains to explain everything in terms that everyone can understand. There is a great temptation to simply get on with the job, build the centre and present a fait accompli: to say, in effect, take it or leave it. The trouble is, there is always that choice, and the choice might fall on the latter alternative. It may be difficult for doctors to return to separate practice premises if they are not enamoured of the health centre, but it is rarely impossible. But they can 'leave it' in other ways too. People can remain in the centre, but without enthusiasm for it. They can work in it, but refuse to take advantage of the opportunities it offers. The health centre would operate, but it would fail to achieve anything like its full potential. It would not be as good as it could be.

Causing the Sap to Rise

Some people expect too much from health centres. They anticipate luxurious premises with facilities approaching those of the local District General Hospital. But there are probably many more who expect too little from them: who contemplate a move into health centre premises with indifference or apprehension: who can see no good coming out of it.

Moving into a relatively large, health authority-owned building, shared with many others, can easily give members of a practice team a sense of being 'taken over': of being submerged, of losing their individuality. They may resent the health centre as something that is being 'imposed' upon them. And, of course, a majority of the people who find themselves working in a health centre may have had no wish to do so. The move may indeed have been imposed upon them, against their will. It is surprising how few people have any real choice in the matter.

The GPs do have relative freedom to decide for themselves. If they do not like the health centre, they can usually threaten to withdraw from it, and make the threat seriously. But even amongst their ranks, there can be a measure of compulsion. Some doctors, it must be said, join the slow migration into shared, purpose-built premises, because they can hardly afford to maintain their own premises, not because of any passion for health centres in their own right. Some are giving up old, decaying surgeries, which either require a lot of money to bring them up to scratch, or are, uncompromisingly, marked down for demolition. Bank managers and bulldozers can seem quite compelling; enough to force an unwanted move into a health centre. But there can be other compelling reasons too. A member of a group practice can simply be out-voted by his partners on the matter, and go along with the majority decision out of an unwillingness to split the group. Quite often, an older doctor will agree to move into a health centre for the sake of a younger and more enthusiastic partner. In at least one case of the latter type the young GP concerned left the practice shortly before the centre opened, and left his senior contemplating a move for which he had never had any liking, and for which he now had no justification.

The doctors' reception and secretarial staff rarely—very rarely—are given any say in deciding whether or not the practice should remove to a health centre. As employees of the doctors, they are almost invariably expected to go along with the doctors' decision, or find other jobs. Rather than work in a health centre, some will indeed look for other work. Many more, especially if they have worked for the practice for some years and are loyal to 'their' doctors, will accept the decision to move even if they are unhappy about it. Practice nurses are in a similar position, as are health authority home nurses, health visitors and midwives. In order to avoid working in health centre premises, health authority nursing staff might at best have to end happy and effective practice attachments. If their senior officers are not willing to be flexible, in common with other health authority employees, and social workers, they might have to choose between the health centre and the sack.

The decision to go into a health centre can seriously threaten the integrity of a primary health care team. Unanimity amongst all the members at the outset is a precious thing, and like most precious things it tends to be uncommon. There are likely to be some who disagree; who would prefer to stay as they are. If feelings are strong enough, people may be willing to give up their jobs, and the disintegration of the team will be literal. More probably, practice team disintegration will be of the insidious type. No-one will consider the health centre issue sufficiently serious to justify resignation, but apprehension about the move, and the sense of disagreement produced, will weaken and disrupt working relationships among team members.

Everyone in the Johnson practice—the three doctors, the three receptionists, and the attached nurse and health visitor—took a pride in how well they got on together. Their relationships with each other were friendly and effective. The shoddiness and decrepitude of their surgery premises hardly seemed to matter. And when the question of moving into a health centre arose, it came as a malevolent and divisive force upon a previously harmonious scene.

Dr Ball, the youngest of the three GPs, was the first to recommend the move, and, to everyone's surprise, he soon managed to convince Dr Johnson himself of the desirability of transferring to a health centre. The youngest of the receptionists was also converted, but Ball did not succeed in convincing anyone else. Dr Green, the third partner, remained quietly hostile to the proposal, and the other four female members of the team were equally hostile and rather less quiet. Inevitably, however, the change was made, and when it was made, Dr Johnson was dismayed and puzzled by the change which came over 'his' practice team.

Rather than comprising one single happy whole, they had gradually split into two distinct 'sides', decided by attitude to the health centre. The two older receptionists, the nurse and the health visitor, were manifestly cool towards Johnson and Ball, and, on occasion, positively unco-operative. When these doctors eventually received their mid-morning coffee, they often found that it was too cold, or contained too much sugar, or too little milk. The receptionists were also less efficient than they had been, because they were not working together as well as they had done. Having quarrelled over the matter of the health centre, they found that they could quarrel over just about anything, and spent large parts of the day so doing. If the youngest of them received a message, there was no guarantee that she would pass it on to her two colleagues; if she needed help, she could not bank on getting it.

Dr Green, for his part, remained in his own room whenever he was in the health centre, spending little time in conversation with his partners. Someone laughingly suggested that he had gone back to working on his own. But, in reality, it was no joke.

Dealing with this dreadful malady of insidious disintegration is really a matter of cure rather than prevention. The only prophylactic is to give everyone in the practice team a veto. And this, of course, is not going to happen, except in rare and unusual cases. There can be very few GPs who would be willing to allow a single receptionist or nurse, or even all the receptionists and nurses, to settle the matter for them.

But to cure the problem requires an understanding of why some people are unhappy about working in a health centre.

There are two principal reasons. The first of these is peculiar to general practitioners, and is that historically-based fear of a health authority takeover.

The second principal reason can exist in the mind of any member of the practice team, for loyalty to the practice is by no means restricted to general practitioners. There are many receptionists and attached nurses and health visitors who contemplate a proposed move into health centre premises with considerable disquiet because they are convinced that the practice will inevitably lose its identity as a result. Unless they are reassured, when the move is completed they will probably discover that they were right. They will see what they have all along expected to see, because that is the way human perception seems to work. Instead of making the best of their new premises, they will make the worst of them. Instead of looking forward, they will constantly be looking back, and the past will seem rosier than it ever did when it was present. Of course, in most health centres they will be right. The centre will indeed be a threat to the identity of the practice team. But even if it is not, even if it is designed specifically for the primary health care team (see the following chapter), initial suspicion and distrust can easily prevent awareness of what might seem obvious fact. The best health centre can accommodate people who see it as a disaster; who are incapable of seeing its virtues and exaggerate its defects, because their vision is distorted by prior conviction of what the health centre must be like—by prejudice, if you like. So it is important to reassure them before the building comes into operation, that their fears are appreciated but are groundless. Similarly with the GPs who suspect an ulterior motive. An excellent way for the health authority to demonstrate that it is interested in working in co-operation with the doctor, rather than in trying to take him over, is to actively involve him in the planning of the health centre.

For all those who are unambiguously against the health centre, there will be many more who could not care less either way: who will come in if they have to, but do not expect it to make any difference to their way of working and furthermore do not want it to. They will be happy to be left alone, will see no need to interfere with anybody else, and consequently will consider themselves to be the very opposite of a problem. From their point of view, their lack of enthusiasm will seem a positive virtue. But they do represent a problem all the same. If the health centre is occupied by people who cannot or will not see its advantages and therefore will not make the most of them, it might as well never have been built. It would have been better to leave each practice in its own separate, up-dated and improved premises. An important part of the pre-opening stage of any health centre must, therefore, be education, or, if you prefer, propaganda. Those who are committed to the health centre must demonstrate to all those who are not just what can be achieved. They have to 'sell' the health centre. They have to demonstrate to all those who do not care, that this is going to be their health centre too: that they can contribute to, and can gain from it. They can flatter them with the true statement that their experience and opinion are of value in the planning of the centre. They have to involve them in that planning process, and in this respect it is not enough to simply invite everyone to the meetings and be delighted when the most notorious awkward sods decide to stay away. The lukewarm and the manifestly cold are not going to come to meetings to discuss the health centre unless they are given a great deal of encouragement. And they should come, so that encouragement should be given.

All in the Same Boat

The aim is a health centre in which all the medical and ancillary participants gain something from each other, enjoy working together in the same building, and share a sense of common responsibility for the development of the health centre and the services it provides. Their interest should not be restricted to their own practice, or their own little segment of the centre. They should be thinking about the centre as a whole, about ways in which it could be made better. In order to make the most of the premises they have been provided with they have to feel that this is their health centre, and that its success is dependent upon their combined effort. Its success is dependent upon their recognising that they are all in the same boat, and if the boat is going to go anywhere, they have to agree on where they want it to go and then co-operate to get it there. Otherwise, it will drift around for ever.

Involving everybody in planning the health centre is a good way of getting them to recognise that they have a shared responsibility for it. But, in practice, the planning process rarely achieves this. Often it actually introduces divisions, and creates or exacerbates a sense of mutual antagonism. It sometimes happens that just a small section of the intending health centre population manages to impose its wishes upon the design, probably because it has been particularly vocal, insistent, and energetic. Where this does happen, it is all too easy for those who do not exercise influence, who do not obtain information about the centre and its progress, and who do not care sufficiently to make the effort, to be suspicious of those who do. For example:

There is a health centre which has been divided right from the start. The two practice groups which occupy it are very different in both style and temperament. The first group consider the second to be old-fashioned, incompetent, unimaginative and politically naive. The second group consider the first to be conceited, intolerant, unaware of their own limitations, and rude. They do not like each other.

They never would have liked each other. They should not be in the same health centre. But they might at least have settled down to a state of

38

quiet disharmony if things had not happened as they did before the centre opened. What happened was that the first group of doctors (the conceited, intolerant, etc., lot) decided that they were going to have their own way. They started to make demands. This came as something as a surprise to the health authority who hoped to get on with the job of planning the centre uninterrupted by petty interjections from intending tenants. But surprise is always a good tactic, and the health authority capitulated to the extent of giving the first group of doctors everything they wanted. However, having had to accede to one group, they took the view that allowing the second group to have their say too would only make their own position twice as bad. Having to contend with four doctors had been bad enough; they were not going to have to deal with eight if they could help it. And the second group made it easy for the health authority to ignore them. They knew what the others had achieved, but did not feel sufficiently interested or confident to insist on equal treatment. They kept quiet and kept to themselves, developing a growing fear that the four conceited GPs were in league with the health authority to do them down. Suspicion and resentment flourished in their breasts. When the health centre opened, they hated it. They felt that their accommodation was nowhere near as good as that provided for the other group, and that nominally common areas of the centre had been taken over by that group with the tacit approval of the health authority. There were many parts of the building which they did not dare to go into. After a month they decided to leave, but changed their minds when they realised that this might be what the others had all along wanted them to do. So they determined to stay, and stick it out. They are still there: permanently unhappy and permanently paranoid. Every suggestion made by the enemy (GPs or health authority) is rejected, even if it seems a good idea on the face of it, because they know they must be up to something. And the doctors in the other group (dedicated to improvement and increased efficiency) get more and more annoyed because, as they see it, the old-fashioned four are vetoing developments out of a dedication to reaction and sheer straightforward awkwardness. Far from being in league with the health authority themselves, they feel that the authority share the attitudes and failings of the opposing group, and use the opposition of the latter as an excuse for their own unwillingness to make any more concessions to them. The caretaker is fond of saying that someday someone will murder somebody. He seems to find the prospect pleasurable.

With two such practice groups it is hard to imagine even the most tactful handling of the planning process having much success in distilling a spirit of partnership and shared enthusiasm for their health centre. Even where the differences are not so great, it is by no means always easy to avoid large-scale conflict and disagreement and to create consensus and co-operation to such an extent that the health centre design and its intended style of operation are accepted unanimously. When a health centre is in being, handling disputes among its participants and encouraging them to reach common decisions can call for considerable skill, and there is much to be said for having a health centre manager who can be responsible for one or a small number of centres. Consideration of health centre management must wait for a later chapter*, but it is worth pointing out here that management of an operating health centre is (or should be) just a continuation of the management of its planning process: the same people have to be brought together, their differences reconciled, their areas of agreement developed. Therefore it makes sense to involve the health centre manager in the scheme more or less from the outset. He can be given the responsibility of ensuring that everybody knows what is going on, encouraging all who expect to work in the centre to participate in its planning, helping to arrange meetings and organise the election of representatives, and generally playing the popular modern role of trouble-shooter. If he is any good at his job, and if other circumstances are propitious, he will so gain the respect and acceptance of all who will be working with him in the health centre long before they move into their new premises, and he will encourage the development of that desired sense of unity and shared responsibility for the future of the centre. If circumstances are not propitious, he will find himself confronted by a collection of people who are so incompatible that no-one could reconcile them.

The more that people are involved in the work of planning their health centre, the more it may become evident that they want quite different things, do not like each other, and would find occupying the same building a far from enjoyable experience. It is better to discover this at an early stage rather than

* Chapter 7.

40

when everyone is committed and has gone to the trouble of moving into the completed centre. This is another advantage of involving in the planning process everyone who intends to work in the health centre: it gives the members of each practice group an opportunity to find out if they will be able to get on with everybody else who will be in the building, and, if not, to consider whether they would be better off joining another, later, health centre in the town, or if that alternative is not available to them, even staying in their own separate practice premises.

The Practical Objections

The way in which the planning process is handled has a lot to do with determining to what extent the health centre will provide value for money. It can greatly influence—one way or another—the motivation of the medical and ancillary personnel to develop more effective working relationships with each other, and it can also influence the extent to which the health centre makes it easier or more difficult for them to work as they would like to do. But despite all the reasons in favour of making the planning process truly democratic, most health authorities are prepared to make only the most grudging moves towards this. Accepting that they have to consult with the various professional interests concerned with the health centre, they will interpret this in the narrowest possible way. They may insist on one GP acting as spokesman for all the other doctors involved, will assume that all health authority employees who will be working in the health centre are represented entirely by their appropriate senior officers, and will never trouble to talk to individual receptionists, or nurses, or health visitors, or social workers. Information about the progress being made will be given to a restricted few, probably at irregular and infrequent intervals, and probably with little explanation or detail. Why is this so?

Many administrators would argue that so abbreviating demo-cracy saves time, and therefore money. The fewer people who are involved, the less argument there inevitably is, and the sooner decisions are thereby made. Small committees get things done. But one must ask, what things? Saving a few weeks or months does not save money if unnecessary faults are incorporated in the design, and if they have to be put right once the health centre is completed. A centre which fails to improve, or even worsens, the quality of primary health care delivery can hardly be said to provide value for money, whatever its initial cost may have been. But to some extent, this talk of saving time is just a health authority excuse. The practical objections to democratic planning are largely red herrings.

Doctors, on the whole, do not like health authorities: they generally regard them with contempt and distrust, they are suspicious of administrators and bureaucrats. They always have been. And there are many health administrators who are none too fond of doctors either, considering them to be far too arrogant and independent, deliberately difficult and preoccupied with their own selfish interests. Of course, there will be many administrators and GPs who do not see each other in such negative ways, but unfortunately there are not more. Antipathy of this kind often has a lot to do with a health authority's failure to encourage GPs to take a full and active part in the planning and design of the health centre they will ultimately be working in. Where doctors are involved to any appreciable extent, this is often because they are seen to have power, and have threatened to use it. In practice, a health authority's attitude on who it is and is not prepared to allow a voice in the planning process is frequently determined by its assessment of the distribution of power: who it feels compelled to listen to, who it feels it can safely ignore.

Usually the only group which has appreciable bargaining power is the GPs. Their power lies in their independence. If they do not like the way a health centre project is developing, it is often possible for them to pull out of it altogether. Sometimes it is easy for the health authority to find a replacement group—there may be plenty of local doctors eagerly waiting for an opportunity to come in. But if a health centre is being planned to include all of a town's doctors, and a good number of them threaten to withdraw, the health authority is going to find it very hard not to give them what they want. The actual amount of power which the doctors have therefore depends—as it does

42

in all industrial disputes—on the ease with which they can be replaced, and the extent to which they present a united front. But most of the people who will be working in the health centre are assumed to have no power at all.

Receptionists and secretaries are under the authority of the doctors, and the health authority may even plan to take them into its own employment when the health centre is built. Most of the others concerned will already be employed by the health authority, and therefore not in much of a position to make demands to it. Social workers, if any are to be included in the centre, have their own senior officers to make the decisions for them.

The health authority may feel happy to ignore nine out of ten of those connected with a centre, because it does not see how they can ever be in a position to threaten it. It can build the centre regardless of their wishes or opinions. But getting the health centre built is not the end of the matter. Presumably the health authority wants its centre to be a success, not simply a construction. And the humble receptionist and nurse have a surprising amount of power when it comes to deciding just how much of a success, or failure, the health centre turns out to be.

The horse can always be transported to the river, but getting it to drink is often a different matter altogether. There are many people who can be taken into a health centre whether they like it or not, but once there, they cannot be compelled to put the building to the uses for which it was really intended. If they feel that the health centre has been imposed upon them, they are unlikely to be enthusiastic about it. They are unlikely to be concerned about exploiting the centre to develop new and better ways of doing things. They are more likely to be preoccupied with re-establishing the old ways. So if being allowed to have a proper say in the planning is dependent upon the possession of power there can be no justification for restricting participation to a few. Virtually all who work in a health centre have power over its fate, and they exercise that power every day, whether they are aware of it or not.

It is undoubtedly true that most nurses and receptionists do not demand their own say on the health centre in which they will eventually be working, and there are many doctors who show a similar lack of interest. And no doubt it will be argued that if people do not want to participate in the planning, there is little point in inviting them so to do. But sometimes it is an invitation that they are waiting for.

An apparent lack of interest may stem from an assumption that such interest would not be welcomed. It may also stem from a belief that the planning stage is a pure formality, because a health centre is a health centre and there is little scope for variation. This latter belief seems to be quite widespread, and if it was corrected, rather more people would presumably be eager to take a part in deciding what sort of health centre was going to be built. Few general practitioners, and even fewer among the other professional and occupational groups involved, seem to know much about health centres, and about alternative designs. Their contact with others who are working in health centres is usually limited or non-existent, so they do not have an opportunity to learn from the happy or unfortunate experiences of others. They do not know what to ask for, they do not know if it is even reasonable to ask for anything, and consequently they can easily be fooled by an administrator or architect anxious to get on with the job. They can be kept quiet with the assertion that such and such a feature is expressly forbidden by DHSS, or has been found to be impracticable or unnecessary elsewhere, or is architecturally impossible. Many believe that it is in the health authority's interest that doctors and everyone else should remain in a state of ignorance, because it is when the masses are educated that they start making demands and holding up progress. But it should be clear by now that the health authority's interest requires that all who are going to work in a centre know, and have plenty of opportunity to say, what they want, if that interest lies in having health centres which not only exist, but which also produce an improvement in the delivery of primary health care. Therefore the health authority has a duty to itself to ensure that all concerned with one of its health centre projects are well informed about the kind of choices available, and about the solutions which have been adopted effectively and ineffectively elsewhere. It is invariably a good idea to arrange trips to other health centres, because they have considerable educational value, and because they can have other benefits too. A few crates of ale loaded in the back of the coach, and kindly donated by the area HA, can do a lot to promote

44

goodwill and create a spirit of camaraderie.

Lack of time can either be a good reason or a good excuse for not wanting to get involved in planning meetings, and which depends often on your point of view. It is easy to be sympathetic towards the doctor who has little spare time because he is devoted to his patients, less sorry where the doctor's devotion is to his golf clubs, but sympathy really should not come into it. The important thing is to get everyone involved, and if there are some who are unwilling or unable to devote much in the way of time to participating in the planning of their new health centre, others have to make the necessary effort to ensure that the time costs of such participation are minimised for them. This means that the health authority, and colleagues who are committed to the health centre and who do want it to be a success, will have to organise things so that they can be involved without having to go to a great deal of trouble. A health centre manager, if he is appointed more or less at the beginning of the project, can shoulder a lot of the responsibility for arranging meetings, ensuring that everyone knows when and where meetings are to be held, reproducing and sending out minutes, and so on. But much of the burden is inevitably going to fall upon the shoulders of (say) the doctor, the nurse, the receptionist who are accorded, and who are prepared to accept, the honour of representing their colleagues in the final tier of planning meetings. Sometimes their duties are so onerous, so expensive in both time and energy, that it is surprising anyone is prepared to take them on. But when a passionate belief in the health centre is not enough to sustain them, self-satisfaction and pride of leadership often are.

There are still going to be people, naturally, who will not be involved in the planning and designing of the health centre they expect to move into, however easy things are made for them, however much they are encouraged, however much they are told that they have a contribution to make. Of course, there are going to be such people. But their failure to be involved should always be seen as a failure by the health authority, by the health centre manager, and by their colleagues who are taking part themselves. It should never be contemplated with satisfaction, or relief, or even indifference. However much effort is made, there are still going to be people who look forward to moving into health centre premises with no particular joy, and who will threaten to hold the centre back from realising its full potential. But if much effort is made, there will be considerably fewer of them than there would otherwise have been.

CHAPTER FOUR

Drawing the Lines

It is largely taken for granted that the justification for health centres lies in their ability to foster the development of a team approach to community care, and help to break down barriers between professions and services. It is surprising, therefore, how inadequate and unimaginative most health centre designs are in this respect. Perhaps too many people assume that simply providing common premises is enough to ensure an improvement in working relationships; that it does not matter how the internal layout is arranged, as long as an all encompassing roof is provided. But in most cases, the roof does little more than keep the rain out, and, sometimes alas, it does not even do this very effectively. What really counts is the way in which the rooms and circulating areas beneath are located. A good design can indeed do a great deal to encourage improved liaison and communication. At best, a bad design leaves things as they were; it can all too easily disrupt existing relationships and create fresh barriers. In terms of working relationships within and across practice team lines, it should never be assumed that the provision of a health centre will inevitably make things better. Without careful thought about the design, it can make things substantially worse.

All too often, it seems, the design work proceeds without proper consideration or appreciation of the aims of the health centre. This often occurs because those aims are not set out clearly, or are confused. This is particularly likely to occur when the people who will actually be working in the centre do not participate fully in the planning of their new premises. Where members of the actual practice teams concerned are not closely involved in developing the design, it sometimes appears easy for health centre planners and architects to forget that separate practice units are in fact going to operate within the centre, and that their maintenance as separate units is indeed desirable.

Although the concept of the health centre is so frequently linked with that of the primary health care team, a health centre design which provides specifically for separate practice-based teams is something of a rarity; the common variety gives the impression of having been planned on the erroneous assumption that the centre would, or should, operate as an undivided functioning whole. This is not to say, of course, that individual practice teams should be provided with total physical isolation, or that the design should not reflect the need for closer liaison between practice teams, and between individual teams and the other services provided in the centre. The layout adopted should be compatible with both these aims: providing for the identity and integration of each of the practice teams, and at the same time encouraging team members to develop more effective working relationships encompassing the health centre as a whole.

In any health centre, however it is designed, the number of people who can be placed in close proximity to each other is severely limited: most people have to be relatively far apart. A room layout which scatters team members throughout the building, and sprinkles other individuals in between, only damages the practice team, and does nothing to encourage wider working relationships. It therefore makes sense to locate all the team members in the same part of the building. Because they work (or should work) closely together, and require frequent contact, they must be given physical proximity. The relative distance of other practice teams, or people providing other services in the centre, will be unlikely to deter the more occasional contact which is being aimed at. If a GP decides that there are advantages in his working more closely with the chiropodist, he is unlikely to be discouraged by the fact that the chiropodist happens to be located at the opposite end of the building. He will be prepared to make the occasional walk or to meet in the common room.

Designing a good health centre therefore means designing for the practice team, and success or failure here generally hinges on what is done in the following four areas: (i) reception and waiting facilities, (ii) accommodation for attached home nurses and health visitors, (iii) the provision of somewhere for the practice team to meet as a team and (iv) the use of decor to help preserve the separate identity of the practice. Each of these will be considered in turn.

One for All or One for Each?

In the vast majority of health centres which include more than one practice, only a single, shared reception area, with its attached waiting area, is provided. In fact, the provision of a common reception area, which serves also as an office and houses the records has become for many people a taken-for-granted feature of health centre design. Occasionally, this area may be partitioned to give separate space for each of the practices, but usually it is not (Fig. 1). Less common variants include separate but linked reception areas serving a shared waiting area (Fig. 2), shared reception but separate waiting areas (Fig. 3), and even separate reception and waiting areas with a single room providing a joint office and housing all the records elsewhere in the building (Fig. 4). But the most radical departure from the norm has occurred in some of the largest centres where each practice has been allocated a particular sector of the building, and given independent accommodation for all these functions (Fig. 5).

Key: R—reception   C—consulting etc   W—waiting

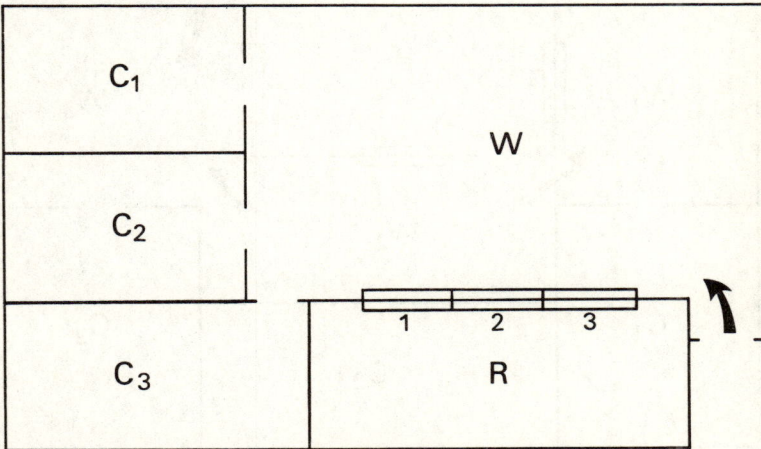

Figure 1 Diagram representing centralised reception/record/office area and associated waiting area

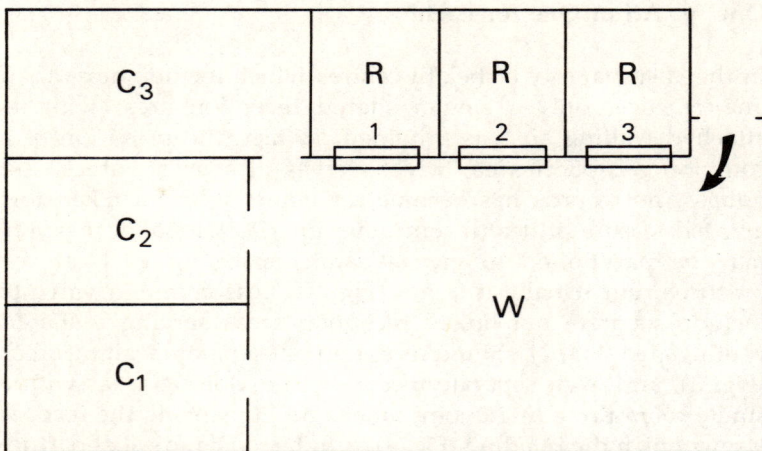

Figure 2 Separate reception/records/office areas, with centralised waiting area

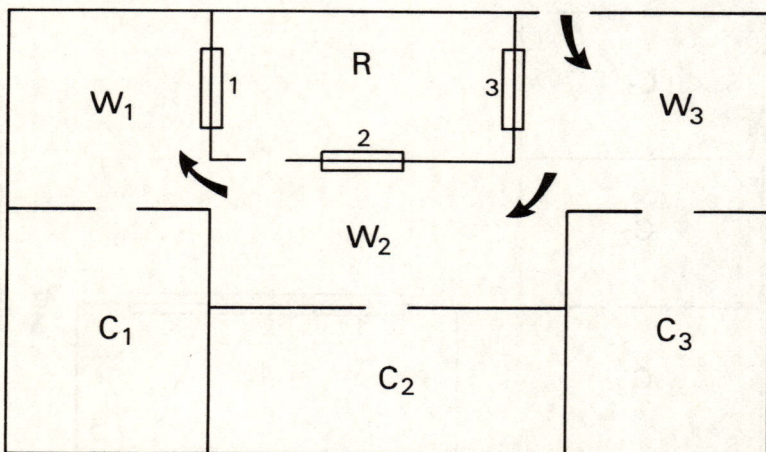

Figure 3 Centralised reception/records/office areas, with separate waiting areas

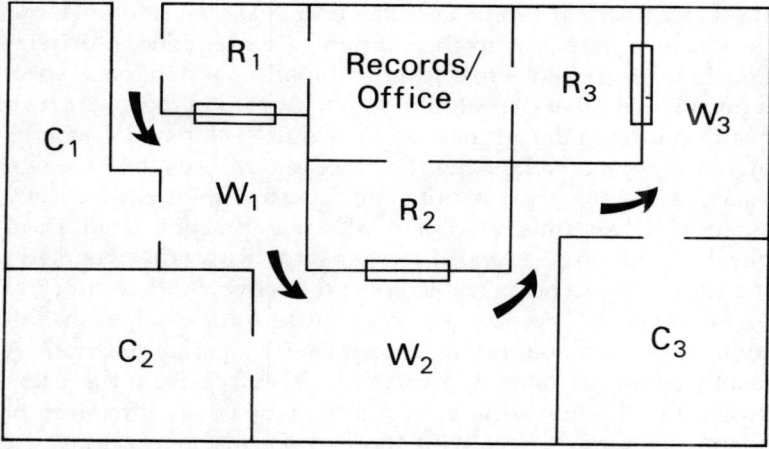

Figure 4 Centralised records/office space, with separate reception and waiting areas

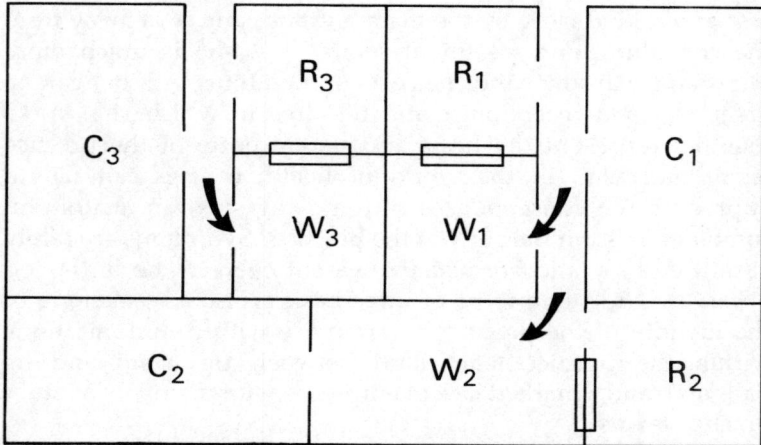

Figure 5 Separate reception/records/office and waiting areas

Clearly, there are some advantages in all these solutions, but the concern here is with their different consequences for relationships inside and across team boundaries, and in this respect it must be said that the solution so far adopted in the majority of health centres is the wrong one. Providing each practice with its own reception area housing the office and records, and its own attached waiting area, is not simply desirable—it is practically essential if an integrated and effective practice team is to develop and survive, and if relationships with other people in the centre are to be amicable and productive. And contrary to popular belief, this is not simply true of the larger health centres, accommodating five, six or seven separate practices. A health centre of only two practices faces precisely the same problems, though admittedly there may be a difference of degree, and must deal with those problems in precisely the same manner.

The liberties taken with the receptionist or secretary and her domain in planning the layout of the centre, stem largely from a failure to appreciate her vital role in the practice team. The function she performs is often equated with that of the caretaker—necessary but peripheral to the main work of the medical professionals whom she serves. On this assumption, she can be physically removed from the rest of the team with impunity, and there is an obvious logic in locating her with the rest of her kind close by the main entrance and well away from the consulting and treatment rooms. But she is much more important than this, and the costs of meddling with her can be great. A good receptionist and the area in which she works together represent the heart and nerve-centre of the practice team, and who in the world of health centres can fail to appreciate the consequences of removing such an anatomical combination from the body of the practice? Symptoms are rarely absent entirely and are usually evident even to the untrained observer. They tend to be of three basic types: a weakening of the identity of the practice, interference with communications within the practice team (and between the team and its patients), and a marked lack of enthusiasm for members of other practice teams.

The identity of a practice team is a difficult thing to define or describe. To some extent it is a matter of the visibility of the team to the patient, and the ease with which it can be distinguished from the rest of the health centre. The patient is not concerned with who employs whom, or who is attached to whom—he judges on the basis of what he sees. And if he sees doctors, nurses, health visitors and receptionists dispersed over a large part of the centre, he will assume that their relationship is not of the closest. To a great extent, the degree to which a practice team is created from a collection of individuals depends upon the degree to which it is recognised and accepted by the patient as a team. It is difficult for them to work together in an effective, co-ordinated manner, if the patient insists on always seeing the doctor, and refuses to be dealt with by the health visitor or nurse. Therefore, it is important that the team should be visible to the patient as a separate, distinct entity, and since the average patient spends the greater part of his time in the health centre being attended to at the reception counter and sitting in the waiting area, the provision of separate such facilities for each practice can go a long way towards achieving this.

Furthermore, the provision of separate waiting and reception areas for each practice greatly facilitates the achievement of that 'domestic atmosphere' which is so frequently declared to be essential for a satisfactory health centre, but which is so rarely achieved. These areas can be comparatively small, and the all too familiar scaled-down version of the hospital out-patients' waiting room can be completely avoided. Instead of row upon row of seated humanity silently contemplating an opposing row of receptionists perched on stools like whores at a bar, or, as in one case, studying the traffic in and out of the lavatories, Mrs Smith can, if she so wishes, pass her waiting time gossiping with Mrs Brown across the reception counter, and not have to strain her larynx in order to be heard. Children seem to be better behaved too when confined in a more limited area, and their parents seem more inclined to exercise control over them. Relatively large waiting areas seem to provide that sense of anonymity which encourages the less restrained patients and their off-spring to indulge in some of the more offensive and bizarre brands of behaviour.

Practice team identity is not only a question of how things look from the patient's point of view, however. Of at least equal importance is the extent to which *the members see themselves* as comprising a discrete unit within the centre, with their own private physical space. And the reception area is of greater significance in this respect than any other room in the health centre. It is of such significance because, unlike the doctor's consulting room, or the nurse's treatment room, it 'belongs' to everybody in the team. Doctors, nurses, health visitors, receptionists, all have a right to be there. It therefore represents the physical centre—the heart—of the practice team. If the team is forced to share it with others, it becomes that much more difficult for them to retain a sense of common identity.

The reception area, and the receptionists themselves also represent a centre of communications for the practice team: not only the formal communications between members necessary to getting the job done, but also the informal, casual contact without which no team ever develops or survives. When the reception area is shared between two or more practices, contact within the team, and especially informal contact, frequently suffers.

The Seacliff Health Centre houses three practices comprising eleven GPs altogether. For reasons already discussed, none of these doctors was very much involved in the development of the design, and their receptionists were frequently to be found smiling loyally, and saying 'what's good enough for the doctors . . .'. In each of the practices, doctors and receptionists got on well together and had worked together sufficiently long for them to know each other's idiosyncrasies. They were fond of describing themselves as 'just like a family', and the exaggeration was understandable. When they discovered that a single, not so large reception area was going to have to do for all three practices, they saw no real cause for concern because they were confident that 'nothing will change. Everyone is so friendly'. But when the health centre came into operation things did not remain the same. The change was subtle, but it was real, and it was generally agreed that it was for the worse.

Right from the start, all but a few of the GPs came into the reception area only reluctantly, briefly, and infrequently. Dr Foster admitted that 'I don't like going in there with all those women. I find it embarrassing'. He came in only when he had specific need, and he left as soon as he could. He did not stay to chat to 'the girls' like he used to do when they were in their old premises. And the receptionists could not help but notice it. Soon they were complaining that 'the doctors are not as friendly as they were, they don't talk to you like they used to'. Even Dr Johnson, who was reasonably thick-skinned, said that he preferred to avoid going into that part of the health centre altogether, because he was afraid of his conversation with 'his' receptionists being overheard by others, or of being way-laid by 'some of the girls with the other practices', who were not his 'cup of tea'. Dr White simply insisted on the receptionist coming to him, quoting his arthritis as an excuse. It was a long way from the consulting rooms to the reception area, which is what the receptionists thought too. One or two of them became quite preoccupied with their feet, and tiredness sometimes strained their loyalty. Now they were frequently to be found baring their teeth and muttering 'Oh hell, he doesn't want me to go down there again, does he?'

So it was that the telephone became everybody's favourite. What started off as a simple novelty, used as much for amusement as anything else, rapidly became venerated as essential to life. People began to wonder how they had ever managed without it. But talking by telephone was nowhere near as much fun as the real thing. Perhaps necessary messages were communicated effectively enough, on the whole, but conversing via a lump of plastic seemed to discourage informality. Dr White rarely got around to asking Aggie about her bad back, and Aggie decided that he must not be interested in her welfare any more. She could not have cared less about his arthritis. Everyone felt just that bit isolated, and it was often said that 'we're not as close as we used to be'. Consequently, although the work did get done, it did not always proceed as smoothly as it might have done, because, for example, the receptionist did not always feel motivated to make things as easy for the doctor as possible. She was less inclined to do him any favours, less inclined to put herself out if a problem arose, more inclined to let him sort the damned thing out himself.

Not only did things deteriorate between doctors and receptionists. Old Dr Flood had grown quite attached to his attached health visitor before he moved into the health centre, but now he hardly ever saw her. Accidental meetings in the reception area were rare. Like his colleagues, he spent as little time in there as possible, and so did the nurses and health visitors attached to the three practices. They too found that the atmosphere in that most crowded and noisy part of the building pretty well discouraged 'just hanging about', and talking 'for its own sake'.

55

It seemed incredible, but there it was. Doctors, nurses, health visitors were all in the same building now, and contrary to all the assumptions actually had less contact with each other in most cases. There were other reasons for this, of course, and these will be dealt with later, but that single shared reception area was an important factor.

Seacliff is quite typical because the deterioration in relationships has been so subtle. There have been no dramatic crises, no disasters. The patients are seen, and on the face of it, everybody is happy. It is only when you dig a little deeper that you discover how teamwork has suffered. Seacliff is by no means the only place in which the biggest danger to the practice team is the health centre itself.

The danger to teamwork is often not spotted because the things on which teamwork depends are not appreciated. Take that question of informal conversation. It seems to be such a waste of time: after all, GPs are paid to treat patients, not to discuss the state of the weather with receptionists. Even asking Aggie about her bad back seems to have pretty limited implications for community health. And of course, it is possible to spend too much time in this way. But it is the opposite error which is the most frequent. A little effort can in fact go a long way in creating a team spirit, and the willingness to spend a little time in casual conversation can reap enormous dividends in terms of mutual loyalty and mutual understanding. After all, a team by definition is a close and intimate affair, and always functions better where the members know each other's idiosyncrasies and way of working. A team also depends on trust, and a sense of mutual help rather than mutual indifference, and these are things which are obviously helped by the creation of a friendly and informal atmosphere. Doctors, nurses, health visitors and secretaries cannot be compelled to work closely together, they have to be motivated. If they do not like each other, if they sense hostility or coldness, they will simply not bother. They will trundle along with the minimum of contact and co-operation.

Some practices go so far as organising social functions out of working hours, and this is fine if this is what the members want. But it is not necessary to go to these lengths. A friendly atmosphere depends on an occasional friendly word as much as anything, besides which, most people these days seem to prefer to keep their work and private lives quite distinct, and have no particular desire to spend their leisure time with people they see all day.

Of course the practice team exists for the patient's benefit, and how effectively it does its job depends very much on how effectively it manages to communicate with its patients. Health centre layout—the way in which reception and waiting areas are distributed—might not appear to have much significance here. But in practice it often does. Health centres with single, shared reception and waiting areas frequently experience problems of communication between the GP and the patient, and also between the patient and the receptionist. This was certainly true of the Seacliff centre.

The practice premises which Dr Foster's group used before the health centre opened were an old terrace house with waiting space in what had previously been the front room. The furnishings were meagre, dusty and well-worn but patients, surprisingly rarely complained about this. Most of them said it reminded them of home. The receptionists were crowded into an adjoining cupboard, and the partition wall between this cupboard and the old front-room had a hole knocked in it to serve as a hatch. Most of the space in this reception area was taken up by several tea chests piled on their sides, which contained the patients' records. There was little room for receptionists: when the electric fire or the kettle was switched on, they had to be careful where they sat; and when a vacancy occurred amongst their ranks, it was said that the smallest applicant was almost certain to get the job.

Despite the primacy of this criterion in selecting receptionists, most of the patients found them friendly as well as tiny, and rarely complained of anything approaching draconian treatment. Rather than acting as a barrier between the doctors and their patients, Mrs Small and her colleagues were often able to supplement the information which the doctor was able to extract from the patient himself, because many of the patients simply liked to talk to them. They often told Mrs Small of social problems which they never thought to mention to the doctor, and female patients sometimes used the receptionists as intermediaries with the doctor, to save themselves the embarrassment of having to tell him what was wrong with them. They played Mum to young girls worried about the start of menstruation; and to middle-aged women worried about the end of it, they were middle-aged women with hot flushes of their own. Even though space was so limited, it was easy enough to take the patient into a quiet corner, without any fuss, for a private conversation; and by means of these preliminary consultations they were sometimes able to ensure that the patient revealed more than she might otherwise have done about her worries or symptoms when she actually got to see the doctor.

When the health centre opened, the receptionists were just reception-ists. They found their job less satisfying, and the patients said they had become 'stuck-up' now that they had moved into a 'posher' place. The fact of the matter was, it was very difficult to hold a friendly conversation across a wide counter and through a glass partition. But more than this, the patients were inhibited by the presence of so many other receptionists behind the counter, and so many other patients in the waiting area behind them. As they saw it, there was no way in which they could talk privately to the receptionist, and this was very largely true. There was no door from the reception area directly into the waiting area, and considerable disruption would have been caused if a patient had insisted on speaking privately. At the least, the receptionist would have had to leave her post and walk an appreciable distance, and then she would probably have had great difficulty in finding somewhere quiet for them to talk undisturbed. Consequently, communications between patients and receptionists speedily deteriorated to the necessary minimum.

It was suggested that a separate interview room should be provided at Seacliff where a patient could talk in confidence to a receptionist if he or she so wished. This solution has, of course, been suggested for other health centres, but proved impossible to implement in this centre because there was no suitable room available and the necessary structural alterations would have proved too costly. Even if such a room had been provided, it probably would not have been used anyway. In the old surgery premises, patients were always chatting to receptionists in odd corners, and no-one knew if they were talking about the patient's sex life or the state of the weather. In the health centre, a patient who asked to be seen in the interview room would immediately be identifying herself to the others in the waiting area as having something to hide: hardly the ideal solution when the aim is to avoid embarrassment to the patient.

This problem can only be satisfactorily overcome where each practice in the health centre has its own reception and waiting areas, and everything is on a smaller and more intimate scale. But even here, things have to be deliberately designed in order to ensure that conversation—private, confidential conversation—between the patient and the receptionist is easy and unobtrusive.

There are some receptionists, of course, who prefer the minimum of contact with patients, and who are grateful for the physical barriers which most health centres provide. Some patients certainly can be troublesome, offensive, and occasionally violent. Young children can be a nuisance. But a receptionist has no more right to be segregated from the patient than has the doctor. If she is not prepared to put up with the occasional difficulty, and cannot cope, then she should not be in this job. If she insists on being substantially insulated from the public, she should go and work in a bank.

The provision of a common reception area with its accompanying centralised waiting area can make things difficult for the patients to talk to the doctor too. This is because it is inevitably a rather long way from that waiting area to the consulting room. Having been summoned to the latter, Granny can take a lot of time putting her knitting back in her bag, creaking to the vertical, and doing her three-legged race down lengthy corridors and through intervening doors so difficult to open that they might have been made by a medieval carpenter with thought of siege in mind. The doctor may be able to spend some of this time usefully by writing up the notes of the previous patient, or reading through those of the next one. But, frequently, much of it is wasted, and therefore he begins to demand that something be done to remedy the situation. This usually means putting a few chairs in the corridor outside his consulting room door and thereby creating a pool of patients instantly available. The undesirability of this practice is constantly being asserted, but it happens because no alternative solution appears to be available. Patients sitting outside the consulting room can always hear what is being said outside it, always listen, and always pretend not to. When their turn to be admitted finally comes, they enter quite aware that they are going to be the next five minutes' entertainment for the odd-looking bunch that is still waiting and (unless they are abnormally thick-skinned or exhibitionist) they are consequently

59

encouraged to reduce their symptoms to the most ordinary and least embarrassing. If they are already disinclined to be honest with the doctor, and to say why they have really come—if they would anyway have hidden behind a smokescreen of alternative, respectable disorders—the presence of the undesired audience is likely to frustrate the efforts of even the most skilled of Dr Balint's disciples to get to the truth of the matter. Where each practice has its own reception and waiting areas, waiting patients can be stored sufficiently close to the consulting room to avoid lengthy delays, and yet far enough away to allow doctor and patient to conduct a confidential conversation without having to resort to whispers.

If having to share a reception area and office space with other practices is bad for relationships within the practice team, it can also often be bad for how the members of the team get on with everybody else in the health centre. At party times, people can enjoy being crowded in large numbers into small spaces, but they tend not to prefer it as a way of life. And shared reception areas in health centres are usually pretty crowded places. Where receptionists continue to be employed by separate practice groups, they are usually anxious to demonstrate their own separateness within the common area. They want to mark out their own territory, and in the absence of natural barriers can resort to artificial barriers to accomplish this. There are health centres in which the receptionists of the different practices have insulated themselves from each other by an ingenious use of filing cabinets, metal shelves and potted plants; and there are other centres in which the frontiers exist only in the minds of the various interested parties, but are real enough all the same. Either way, the effect is to impede movement (and worsen tempers) in an enclave which is already sufficiently congested to discourage locomotion and foster frustration. Even when the receptionists start off quite positively inclined towards each other, even when they are inclined to commence with shows of friendliness, after they have had their toes trodden upon a few times—literally or figuratively—their bonhomie becomes a little strained. Crowding creates conflict. So whereas receptionists working in their own autonomous areas spread around the health centre might co-exist quite happily, forcing them together in a single tiny enclave can ultimately be very bad for their—and everybody else's—efficiency and tranquillity.

It is bad enough when the women are in conflict. But whenever women *are* in conflict, they often feel it necessary to involve the men. Disputes between receptionists can quickly become disputes between GPs. Relationships between entire practice groups can easily become soured as a result of tensions and disagreements among receptionists competing for limited working space.

Annie Broom was the sort of woman who likes to run things. She thought she was very good at running things. She thought she had a right to run things. In the old surgery, nobody questioned that. She organised Lily and Jean, her fellow receptionists; and, in many ways, she organised 'her' doctors too. Nobody ever argued with her.

Half a mile away, in the premises of Drs Spencer, Crawford and Ross, Mrs Nutt had had greatness thrust upon her. Insofar as anybody had to, it was taken for granted that Mrs Nutt should take charge, for Mrs Jolly only worked part-time, and Sandra was but a girl.

When the health centre opened, the half-mile shrank to a few feet and disappeared altogether in places, but the people did not change. Annie Broom considered that the entire reception area was hers to govern as she wished. At ten past nine on the morning of the first day, she made Mrs Jolly cry. And when Sandra had been reprimanded for singing, having a dirty overall, and winking at Annie's male patients, it was obvious to Mrs Nutt that things could not go on like this. So far, she herself had escaped Annie's attentions, but she had a responsibility to defend her friends. However, she did recognise that Annie was of too heavy a weight to be tackled by her alone. Therefore she called upon Dr Spencer. He promised that he would have a word with Dr O'Flynn, Annie's employer, and he did. But O'Flynn resented the interference, and said so. There followed a quarrel which was not quickly forgotten.

Conflict, of course, is not inevitable where the receptionists of separate practices are compelled to share working areas, but it is more likely to occur than where each practice has its own autonomous reception and working areas. Where such separate provision does not exist, and particularly where—as is often the case—the space allocated to office and reception functions is cramped and claustrophobic, the possibility of tensions developing, and manifesting themselves in the form of overt disagreement, must be borne very much in mind, and a conscious effort made to avoid trouble, or spot it and deal with it before it has a chance to produce real disruption in the working of the health centre and of each individual practice.

Conflict is not inevitable, and the receptionists of the different practices may even come to realise certain advantages of their working in close physical proximity. They may develop a degree of mutual aid, being prepared to help each other out, to a limited extent, particularly when one group is under strength because of illness or holidays, or at other times of pressure. But such mutual aid, where it does develop, does tend to remain on a very limited scale, and the possibility of its occurring cannot justify providing all the practices in a health centre with a single, shared reception area. The disadvantages vastly outweigh any possible advantages. Even when tensions and hostility do not develop between the different groups of receptionists, it seems to be at least as likely that they will simply maintain a state of peaceful co-existence, isolating themselves from each other, as that they will develop a habit of helping each other out. The most amicable ladies are apparently often willing to sit with little to do, and watch the receptionists of another practice scurrying about madly trying to cope with a crisis with less than their usual complement. Nor is their failure to lend a hand by any means always resented. Indeed, resentment might follow if they *did* offer their assistance. Each practice is invariably anxious to retain its separate identity, and the members of each practice team generally want to be left to get on with their work without anyone from other practices getting involved—even when the going does get rough. Offers of help can easily be interpreted as interference, or as implied criticism of their own efficiency.

Where receptionists continue to be employed by the GPs, and therefore retain primary allegiance to the separate practices in the health centre, they are unlikely to gain much benefit from sharing a common working area. They are going to be disinclined to develop mutual aid on any scale, preferring to retain their own autonomy and not become involved in the affairs of others. They will only come to work together to any extent where they share the same employer—and this means, where the health authority takes over responsibility for receptionists in the health centre, either by taking the doctors' existing receptionists onto its establishment, or by appointing new ones. This question of who should employ receptionists in the health centre is quite a complex one, for each alternative has its pros and cons, and its consideration must therefore be left for another chapter.

Joining the Ladies

The way in which members of primary health care teams are usually dispersed over the area encompassed by the building might lead one to think that the authorities involved did not approve at all of such groups, and had used physical dispersal in order to break them up. There are doctors in one corner, receptionists in another, and attached nurses and health visitors hidden away in a third. Surely somebody must be making a deliberate effort to stop them fraternising as they used to do? At least, that is the impression one gains—that health centres are designed for the purpose of keeping the doctors and the nurses well and truly apart. It is hard to believe that the opposite effect is ever intended.

No doubt it is economical in terms of the direct cost of the building to provide all attached nurses involved in the health centre with a single, shared room, and to do the same for the health visitors or the midwives. Giving each nurse and health visitor a separate room adjoining the consulting rooms of the doctors she works with is going to be more expensive, but if more effective primary health care teams really are desired, this is absolutely essential. The alternative—which has been adopted in most health centres built so far—is bad for the team in two ways: first of all it hinders communications between team members, and secondly discourages team spirit and the sense of actually forming a unit working together for the same ends. The second of these disadvantages might seem the least substantial, but it represents the biggest danger because if team spirit thrives everyone will make the effort to maintain communications whatever the difficulties—if it disappears, everything else becomes irrelevant, because the primary health care team will cease to exist.

Having all members of the practice team simply based in the same building does not guarantee that communications among them will improve. In fact, it does not even make it inevitable that they will remain as good as they were before the practice moved into the health centre. Sometimes things can turn out to be very much worse because the team is worse accommodated than it was in its previous premises.

Drs Stone, Young and Clegg had the sort of enthusiasm that made them keen on the health centre right from the day it was first suggested. As far as they were concerned, it was an opportunity to develop their practice still further, and they had already done quite a lot in this respect. For example, the attachment of a health visitor and a nurse to the practice had been accomplished a couple of years before, and they were all working well together. They were fortunate in occupying a comparatively large house with accommodation on three floors, and there had been no difficulty in finding room for a well equipped treatment centre which was the preserve of the SRN, as well as comfortable offices for herself and the health visitor. One of the attic rooms provided a common-room where the team could meet informally and hold weekly practice meetings. Before the move into the health centre, therefore, communications amongst them were easy and effective, and the very nature of the premises indicated that they were a distinct unit. Drs Stone, Young and Clegg were able to communicate their enthusiasm for the health centre to everybody else in the practice. Health centres they said, were the latest thing, so the move was bound to improve things. That it might make things worse was never countenanced.

The health centre was really an extension of an existing health authority clinic, and quite early on in the project—well before the centre actually came into operation—people got into the habit of describing it in terms of two halves: the GPs' half and the health authority half. The health authority half comprised the old clinic building, and the new bit was assigned to the doctors and their receptionists. The clinic had 'always' provided accommodation for all the nurses, midwives and health visitors working in that part of the town, and it was not considered necessary that separate rooms should be provided for the health visitors and nurses attached to the three practices coming into the health centre. As far as the health authority was concerned, facilities were already provided for them in the clinic building, and therefore, when the health centre was in business they would continue to use those facilities. It meant that they would be at the opposite end of the building from the doctors, but at least they would be in the same building and it did not seem too bad. It would not be all that far to walk and it might even turn out to be easier than climbing all those stairs in the old surgery. What Drs Stone to Clegg did not consider was that there would be lots of other people around in the new premises to get in the way.

Once they were working in the health centre, things deteriorated suddenly and, apparently, permanently. Communications deteriorated in quantity and quality. What that means is that they did not talk to each other as much as they used to do—there were weeks when they hardly talked to each other at all—and when they did talk, it was increasingly over the 'phone and usually brief and very much to the point. They did not work together in the way they had done before. They did their separate jobs separately.

Maybe it is more usual for a practice team to move into a health centre from premises in which there was hardly room for the doctors, let alone anybody else, but even in such cases it should not be taken for granted that GPs and attached nurses or health visitors will see more of each other, and have more opportunity to talk, than previously. Being in the same building can create an assumption that contact will somehow come automatically, and that no-one need make a deliberate effort to ensure that it occurs. Such an assumption could not be made about tiny premises in which there is hardly room for the health visitor or nurse to enter without somebody having to leave through the back door, and certainly no desk, let alone room, of their own. So if people do want to see each other, it they want to work effectively together and discuss things fully, they have to make a deliberate effort. And sometimes they do. Going into a health centre can easily give the impression that no more effort is required: that all the problems are solved, and everyone can take a rest. Now that they all have rooms in the same building, they are bound to bump into each other, or pop in and out of each other's rooms, almost accidentally. Nobody has to try. Dr Black can sit in his consulting room, and take it for granted that Mrs White the health visitor will call in to see him if she needs to, or they will see each other by chance in the corridor. And

Mrs White can sit in the room she shares with all the other health visitors, and make precisely the same assumptions.

When Dr Maple and his colleague Dr Butler had their surgery on Cemetery Road, Mrs Cope the health visitor had been in the habit of calling in at ten o'clock every morning to confer with them. When the last of the patients had been seen, Flo the receptionist would put the kettle on, and Mrs Cope would join the two doctors in Dr Maple's consulting room where they would discuss whatever had to be discussed. A quarter of an hour later, she was—as she was fond of saying—back on the streets again. It did not take up much of her, or anybody else's time, but meeting regularly like this made a big difference to the way they worked together. Then they moved into the health centre. Mrs Cope would join the other health visitors for morning coffee in the common room; Drs Maple and Butler got Flo the receptionist to take them their coffee in their consulting rooms. They did not see each other for days on end. They did not make much effort to, and once they had got out of the habit of meeting, things stayed like that. They all agreed that it was unsatisfactory. They all agreed that something would have to be done about it, but as they kept waiting for each other to do the doing, nothing ever was.

Accidental contact between team members, when they are dispersed over a reasonably large health centre, can be surprisingly infrequent, and when it does occur, there is a fair chance that somebody will not have the time to stand and talk. The closer they are together in the health centre, the more chance they have of meeting without having to make a deliberate effort to do so. But of course, satisfactory contact really does depend upon people making the effort, going out of their way to ensure that they do get together as often as necessary. Having the GPs in the team at one end of the health centre, and the nurses and health visitors at the other, discourages people from making the effort in at least two ways.

Even the largest health centre is not so large that the walk from one end to the other is not feasible—occasionally, at least. So why, for example, do not the doctors perambulate over to the nurses', or the health visitors', room, to engage in a little direct contact? They may have a natural reluctance to move anywhere under their own steam, but there is also the frequently expressed dislike of going into a room in which large numbers of strange women might be found. There *are* doctors who would be reasonably happy to enter a room in which they could be fairly certain of finding a woman they are familiar with quite alone. But having to face maybe half a dozen of the species, most of whom are comparatively unknown would be quite a different matter. A male doctor can find encroaching into a well-populated female stronghold quite an unpleasant experience, and it is not surprising if he decides that the benefits of seeking direct contact are not worth the associated discomfort and embarrassment.

Traffic is still possible in the opposite direction, though. The nurse and health visitor can occasionally leave the sanctuary of their strongholds and seek out the doctors in their own lairs. Sometimes they do, but they do it rather less often than might be expected. The reason why they do it less often than expected brings us on to the second of our major points: the problems physical dispersal of team members creates for team spirit.

There is no doubt about it, the fact that attached nurses, health visitors and midwives remain in the employment of the health authority makes difficulties for the integration of the primary health care team. There are practical difficulties which will be discussed in the next chapter, but over and above these is the effect upon team spirit, the sense of unity. It can be difficult to overcome the feeling that the primary health care team is no team at all, but just an uneasy alliance of people ultimately devoted to different, and frequently opposing, sides. Nurses are conscious of the fact that the health authority pays their wages, and that it is the senior nursing officers, outside the team, who decide what they can, and cannot, do. GPs are aware of this as well, and the awareness often makes it impossible for them to recognise attached nurses as full members of any team to which they themselves belong. In practice, and with luck and under-standing, the fact that the nurses and health visitors are on the health authority side can be half-forgotten as the team members get on with their work free from outside irritation. As long as the fact of health authority control over a good part of the team does not become manifest, its members at least have a chance of putting this fundamental division out of their minds and coming to regard themselves as a unit with their own distinct identity.

One way of making it manifest is for health authority officers to do something which is seen as interference in the working of the practice team. Another way of making it manifest—giving it tangible, physical, immediately visible form—is to put the GPs in a half of the health centre labelled accordingly, and to accommodate team members employed by the health authority in a distinct 'health authority half'. There may be practical, economic reasons why shared accommodation is provided for all health visitors, nurses, midwives based in the centre, but it can also create an impression that when the crunch comes, when a decision has to be made whether they rightly belong alongside the GPs in the practices to which they are attached or lumped together with the other health authority services, then the health authority has no doubts on what that decision should be.

Health centres can affect working relationships in many ways. One way is by appearing to give physical form to certain relationships, or by seeming to discourage other relationships and somehow suggesting official disapproval of them. If a health centre is designed specifically for the practice team—if it provides all members of the team with working space within the team's own autonomous area—then it has enormous value for the morale of the team, for team spirit. It gives members the feeling that what they have achieved, or are trying to achieve, is recognised as being worthwhile, and worth building for. It encourages them to keep on trying. It gives them a pride in what they are doing. If the design divides the team, and scatters it all over the place, the members are going to be less than encouraged. It can hardly be wondered at if they lose enthusiasm for the whole concept of the primary health care team, and simply give up, settling back within the old divisions that the health centre gives tangible form to.

This business of concentrating health authority-employed team members in shared rooms well away from the doctors' consulting rooms is most evident when the health centre is created by expanding an existing clinic. Here, there are already nurses' rooms and health visitors' rooms in existence, and it seems logical to keep them in use when the expanded building comes into operation. But even where there has been an opportunity to plan the health centre from scratch, this particular method of accommodating members of the primary health care team is all too often adopted. Obviously it is cheaper than providing each nurse, health visitor and midwife with her own room. And it can reasonably be argued that if separate rooms were provided, they would be unoccupied for much of the working day. This argument is also used against the provision of individual consulting rooms for GPs in the centre, and there are many (but not many GPs!) who feel that it would be more logical for two or three doctors to share a single room and stagger their surgery hours. Among the several arguments against this, one is crucial: it would seriously damage the separate identity of each practice, and the preservation of that identity is what practice members and patients very much want. But the same applies to the accommodation of the nurse, and the health visitor. Matters of efficiency are rarely as simple as they seem. The task is not to provide a health centre as cheaply as possible; it is to provide a health centre that *does its job properly* as cheaply as possible. This is not going to be achieved by providing facilities for team members which are so dispersed and segregated that their contact with each other, and their very sense of unity, is disrupted. So building a health centre that is a success is going to be more expensive than building a health centre that is a failure—but this applies to most things. In this case, it may not be just a ha'porth of tar that it is involved, but relative to the overall cost of the building, it can come close. The home nurse, the health visitor, and (if there is one) the midwife attached to the practice could share a single room within the practice area, and if only two or three practices are based in the centre, the number of rooms involved is going to be small.

Despite what has been said, it does not always happen that communications within the practice team deteriorate after moving into a health centre where the health authority members of the team are physically segregated from the GPs. Of course, it often applies that simply being in the same building does make it easier for there to be contact between doctors and attached nurses or health visitors. It does not always apply that because contact is *easier, more* contact occurs, but sometimes it does. Things may have been so bad before the move into the health centre that putting all the team members in the same building, however spread out they might be, cannot make them worse, and stands a good chance of making them better. But the intention is not to create health centres that are no worse, or slightly better, than the worst that went before. The intention is to create the best possible health centres, and this means health centres that make contact among primary health care team members as easy as it can be made, and give them such a sense of team identity that they want to communicate and work more closely together—that they are motivated to take advantage of what the health centre makes easy. This means designing for the primary health care team. It means giving each practice its own autonomous area with the health centre: separate waiting and reception areas, and accommodation for *all* team members within the practice area. In addition to this, it means giving the team somewhere to meet as a team.

Common Sense on Common Rooms

Not all practice premises outside health centres are sufficiently commodious to allow all the team to meet together, but surprisingly many are. They may not have a room which can be set aside purely as a common room, and used for such meetings, but they may well have one comparatively large consulting room, or even the waiting room which can be used at certain times for all to get together to discuss patients and the team itself. It does not always follow that where such meetings are physically possible they will in fact take place. Most practice teams do not have them, and show no interest in holding practice meetings in the future. But teams which do not meet together regularly are not going to become real teams—they will exist at a much lower level. They might argue that the work gets done, and the patients get seen, just as effectively without meetings of the whole team, but they are missing the point: they are missing the opportunity to act as a team, and to make team decisions. They are simply working as a series of related individuals. They are failing to apply the range of expertise which they have collectively available to the problems patients present. This does not mean that all problems require consideration by the whole team, but in any practice, in any week, there are bound to be some which would benefit from this. Furthermore, all meeting together as a team is of vital importance in creating and sustaining a feeling of being a team. Apart from having an opportunity to discuss and improve their way of working together, the sheer fact of sitting down and talking together creates a feeling of solidarity that manifests itself with benefit in the day-to-day working of each individual member.

Therefore, if the health centre is to encourage maximum development of the primary health care teams it houses, it has to make it easy for them to meet, separately, as teams. It has to provide somewhere for practice meetings to be held. In the vast majority of cases, it does not. None of the rooms 'belonging' to the practice can be easily given over to such a function: there are no large consulting rooms where all can gather for a weekly meeting. Consulting rooms are designed for a doctor and a patient—that is all. Waiting areas cannot be used. Even where the practice is fortunate enough to have its own waiting and reception areas, this is unlikely to be so closed off from the rest of the centre that a confidential meeting is possible. In most cases, where there is one large central waiting area, the team might as well hold its meeting in the street outside as sit in there. That leaves the common room.

Every health centre has its common room. The common room is considered essential to the aim of producing some overall sense of unity and shared purpose among all those working in the centre. It might conceivably lend itself to the other aim of promoting effective primary health care teams. But the idea of a common room is that it is common, and open to anyone who happens to feel like using it. The only way in which this room can be used for practice meetings is by producing a timetable so that certain groups have exclusive use of it at certain times, and everyone else is banned from entering. Assuming that the different practice teams in the centre did not insist on having their meetings at the same time, this could be done. But it could only be done at the expense of preventing the common room from fulfilling its intended purpose for at least part of each week. This may not be too much of a problem if there are only a small number of groups in the health centre, and the common room will not be out of commission for very long; and in existing health centres where alternative accommodation for practice meetings is not possible, this is the only solution. Holding

71

practice meetings in the common room, and preventing other people from using it for a time, is preferable to not holding practice meetings at all. But ideally the primary health care team should have somewhere of its own to hold its meetings. Having to go to the trouble of arranging for use of the common room and denying everybody else in the health centre access to it may deter team members from getting together at all. If they have a room of their own, there are no such problems.

There are two principal objections to providing each practice in the health centre with its own common room in addition to a large common room for the benefit of everyone working in the centre. The first of these objections is that if the team members can take their ease entirely within their own territory, they will not have contact with people in the building outside their own team, and there will not develop the overall sense of unity, and the improvement in working relationships across practice team boundaries that is desired. This assumes that only having the one common room, for everybody's use, has an integrative effect. But what happens in practice? How often do common rooms attract simultaneously people from all the practices in the centre, together with individuals providing health authority services in the building? How often do they resound to the laughter and conversation of the massed populace? How often are their expensive armchairs entirely occupied? How often are they used at all? There may be cases where the common room is really used as it is supposed to be used, but these are few and far between.

The following is a record of the use to which the common room in one medium-sized health centre was put on a reasonably typical day. Throughout that day, the observer remained in the room or sufficiently close to it to be able to observe the traffic in and out.

Until 10.30 in the morning, there was no such traffic at all. Then a solitary GP opened the door, looked briefly inside and departed again, closing the door behind him. Some ten minutes later, two nurses came in bearing cups of tea. They sat down in one corner of the room, and conversed together in what can only be described as low tones. A young receptionist arrived next. She glanced at the two nurses, took a magazine from a rack by the door, and sat down in the opposite corner of the room. A quarter of an hour later, all three had departed.

72

At just after twelve o'clock, the chiropodist came in, carrying his sandwiches in a Tupperware box. He ate them, and left. Twelve thirty brought a veritable invasion of receptionists—four, to be precise—who divided into two groups of equal size.

Soon afterwards, a doctor opened the door, with the obvious intention of saying something to the ladies in one of these groups. Having seen the ladies in the other group, however, he decided against holding his conversation in the room. He therefore indicated to his own reception- ists that he would like to see them outside. They departed accordingly, and did not return.

From 1.30 until 3.30 the room was empty, but then two individuals entered simultaneously. One was the 'school doctor'; the other, the senior receptionist of the largest practice in the centre. They ignored each other, and drank their coffee in silence. When the man had gone, the senior receptionist asked the observer 'Who was that?' On the date in question, they had both been working in the building for almost exactly two years.

At 4.25 a receptionist looked in, presumably in search of someone. At 5 p.m. the observer went home.

Sometimes one practice group, or a group of health authority personnel, take over the common room, and come to treat it as their own private property.

In one health centre which accommodated two large practices, one group gained the upper hand from the opening day. The common room was large and well furnished. It had a small kitchen attached. The receptionists of the dominant group began by taking over the kitchen. They used it for making morning or afternoon tea or coffee, they used it for preparing lunches, and they made it clear that they had no intention of sharing it with anyone else. The ladies of the other practice were of a comparatively timorous nature, and their fear of confrontation led them to avoid it. They 'made do' with a kettle in the reception area.

For a time, however, the doctors of the 'inferior' group acted as if they had equal right of access to the common room. There were occasions when they actually came and sat in it. But this did not last for very long. Whenever they did come and sit, they invariably found already seated there at least a representative selection of the members of the opposing practice team. And when they entered, the conversation would drop to a whisper, and they would be glared at icily for intruding. At first, they took to knocking before entering, but even this did not seem to satisfy those already occupying the room. Their very presence was deplored.

Eventually, nerves cracked. Such intrusions occurred less and less frequently. The 'dominated' doctors decided that they did not need a common room anyway. It was not as if they wanted to talk to anyone in the other group, or as if anyone in the other group wanted to talk to them. It was easier all round if they simply stayed out of the room altogether. So they did.

Common rooms are often used solely as kitchens, where tea is brewed to be distributed by foot-sore receptionists to waiting GPs who remain in their consulting rooms. Even where the common room is used for its intended purpose, GPs are usually noticeable by their absence, preferring to partake of their refreshment in private. This is often interpreted as an unwillingness on the part of the doctors to mingle with the riff-raff. But there are other reasons.

It frequently happens that keen GPs make a special effort to frequent the common room in the early days of the health centre, and to take their morning coffee with the madding crowd. But even these worthy souls often find that their best intentions cannot survive the pressures of practicality. Therefore, they eventually give up this friendly act, and ask that the receptionist bring their beverage into their own rooms. Sitting at their own desks, they can get on with correspondence and other matters—they can do something manifestly useful, whereas sitting in the common room can seem a waste of time.

So, with time pressing, they conclude that they have better things to do than sit in the common room and make polite conversation to people they have no practical, immediate reason for talking to. And, of course, there are many doctors who keep out of the common room because they simply do not want to have anything to do with people outside their own practice. Some might call it snobbishness, but as it is often other doctors that they are most reluctant to meet, it might be more accurate to call it a preference for the company of people they know—members of their own practice group. Nor is this feeling of wanting to stick to one's own exclusive to GPs—people in every profession and occupation in the health centre can be guilty of it, if indeed it is a crime. Consequently, in practice, common rooms are not always as good as they are supposed to be at bringing everybody in the health centre together. If people are going to meet in a common room, they have to *want* to meet in a common room. Providing a common room, but failing to provide for the identity and effective working of the practice team is a good way of making sure that a large part of the health centre population will not want to meet people outside their own team.

It has to be said again, the vast majority of GPs, receptionists, and attached nurses, health visitors and midwives are much more concerned that their practice should survive intact, than that they should develop wider working relationships encompassing the health centre as a whole. Consequently, if they feel that the identity of the practice is threatened in the health centre, if they see others as interfering and encroaching, they are more likely to be hostile than friendly towards them. Rather than fraternising with them in the common room, they are going to want to shut themselves off from everyone outside the practice team as much as possible. Therefore, providing a large common room for everybody's use is not going to have much of an integrative effect. It does not make much sense, then, to deny each practice team somewhere to meet as a team on the grounds that this would prevent people getting together in the common room! In fact, designing for the primary health care team—and this means giving them somewhere of their own to hold practice meetings—is more likely to encourage them to have more contact with others outside the team. If the identity of their practice is secure, if they can work together without feeling that other people in the centre are getting in the way, they are less likely to become hostile towards them, more likely to appreciate the benefits of developing more effective working relationships with them. If the practice team has somewhere of its own to meet, its members may be more, not less, likely to use the health centre common room, and to enjoy meeting and talking to people outside the team.

The other objection to giving each practice team its own common room is, inevitably, financial. A room which is going to be used, at most, only for an hour or so once or twice a week does not appear to be very cost-effective. So something has to be done in order to give the team a private meeting area without going to the expense of providing a purpose-built room. Having said that waiting areas in health centres—even where each practice has its own—are rarely sufficiently isolated from the rest of the health centre to serve this purpose, there would seem to be a need for architects to come up with schemes for screening off the waiting area in order to allow meetings to be held outside surgery hours. However, this will have to be achieved without obstructing access to the reception counter for those patients coming to make appointments or collect prescriptions.

The Colour Question

The final element of designing for the primary health care team appears the most trivial, and probably is, which is why something at least is sometimes done about it. Perhaps, comparatively trivial as it is, it has appeal to the interests of the architect. This is the question of decoration and furnishing. Now if the practice is to be easily identifiable and distinguishable from the rest of the health centre, an easy way of doing this is to paint it a distinctive colour. This is often done—not always, but often. Sometimes colour differentiation goes no further than the signposts bearing the doctors' names, and it is obviously difficult to go much further than this if the practice is sharing some facilities with other practices, and has its members dispersed in rooms all over the building. But if each practice has its own, comparatively self-contained, area, there is no reason why this cannot be decorated as a unit, distinct from the rest of the centre. This then raises the question of who should choose the decorations. It is rather taken for granted that this must be left to the architect, with perhaps the odd health authority officer making his contribution. But why should the team members not have a chance to choose their own wallpaper and their own curtaining? The colours surrounding us can make a big difference to how we feel in the course of a busy day. Therefore, people in health centres may work that bit more happily if they have had a chance to choose their own decorative environment. It also gives another chance for involvement in the health centre planning, and the virtues of this have already been discussed. Of course, they cannot have a free hand. Somebody has to ensure that the decor is not so idiosyncratic that it clashes with the rest of the building, but a lot can be achieved with a little tactful guidance.

Tact is often needed, but usually lacking, when it comes to selecting furniture. Problems arise when the doctors coming into the centre want to bring with them items from their old practice premises. Sometimes they want to do this purely for sentimental reasons—to maintain a link with what is about to become the past; to reaffirm that things have not really changed, that the practice still exists, that its identity is still intact. Not all will want to do this—there are many who are delighted to be rid of the ancient rubbish they have had to put up with for years, and look forward to some modern stuff at last. Young doctors recently recruited to the practices are naturally likely to be least attached to existing furnishings, most anxious to move into new premises with up-to-date trappings. Older doctors may be ready for a change too, but some of them will not. What should be done? Usually what is done is that they are told by architects and health authority officers that the old is too big to fit in the new, tailor-made consulting rooms, or that it would simply look out of place. This might be true, and with a bit of tactful handling, the GP concerned might come to see this. But if he is insistent, and if there really *is* room for the stuff, however much it might clash with the space-age fittings of the rest of the building, he should be allowed to bring it in. After all, the aim is not to design a building that looks pretty, if this is at the expense of antagonising people who will be working in it, making them feel that their practice has been stripped of its identity, and that the building itself together with everyone else who works in it pose some kind of threat. The need is to encourage commitment to the health centre, and enthusiasm for what it makes possible. Everything has to be handled from the point of view of motivating individuals, not creating an artistic delight.

Sometimes doctors may wish to retain an item of furniture for practical reasons: a chair that somehow seems to ease away lumbar pain, or a desk that can easily accommodate two fat knees. Certain pieces may be quite old and valuable, and if the doctor has nowhere to put them at home—if his wife refuses to have them in the house—and he is unwilling to part with them, taking them into the health centre is his only hope. Some may feel that an elaborately carved bookcase, or an elephantine mahogany desk, improves their status and encourages the right kind of respectful attitude in the patients. Furniture can have practical value in intimidating the patients. One doctor, for example, insisted on bringing into the health centre with him a low couch which was the only seating arrangement provided for his patients in the consulting room. This, coupled with a high chair which he perched himself upon, gave him a considerable height advantage over even the tallest patient. He had a quite pathological preoccupation with his own physical mediocrity, and was anxious to do anything to create a temporary superiority of stature. He seemed to think that without this, the patients would have such contempt for him that he would be quite incapable of doing his job. Cases which indicate a need for psychiatric therapy will probably be rare, however, and most requests to transport furniture or other items from the old premises to the new will have an element of sense in them, if it is looked for. Sometimes the doctor concerned can be convinced that he will be at least as well served by the new items already ear-marked for the centre—hopefully, it should be possible to show him that he will be better off. But the preferences of the people who will be working in the centre must be respected. A feeling that the centre has deprived them of things they valued or cherished or were simply used to, and has replaced them with things inferior, must be avoided.

Allowing the people who will be working in the centre to have a say in how it will be decorated, furnished, and equipped provides another chance to create a sense of involvement in the project, to foster a feeling that this is 'their' health centre, that they are responsible for it, and that it is up to them to make the best use of it. This applies also to the fitting out of rooms occupied by health authority employees. It does not matter that the equipping of the treatment room can be quite effectively planned by a nursing officer who will not be working in that room. By failing to ask the nurse who will be responsible for the treatment room what *she* wants, and what she considers to be necessary, an opportunity will be lost to show her that she really *is* responsible for that room, that what she has to contribute *is* important, and that the health centre is not something that is simply being imposed upon her, but is a new opportunity with which she is directly involved.

Good health centre design means designing for the primary health care team: providing premises in which the team can work together easily as a unit, in which they are easily identifiable as a unit to the patients and to each other, and in which they do not feel themselves to be threatened by outsiders. It is not inevitable that providing such a building will make for more effective, better integrated primary health care teams, nor is it inevitable that team members will in fact come to like other people in the health centre, and actually develop new, or more effective, working relationships with them. Physical surroundings cannot determine these things—what happens depends on other things too, and some of these will be considered in the following chapter. But physical surroundings can make an important contribution, and every effort must be made to ensure that they facilitate and encourage, rather than hinder and discourage, the best possible working relationships.

CHAPTER FIVE

Chiefs, and Chiefs and Indians

The Heavyweight Contest

Regrettable as this may be to some, the health centre has no single boss, nor, for that matter, has the primary health care team. There might be some individuals who would like to occupy that position themselves, or who even like to think that they already do so. But, in reality, no single person can exercise authority over everyone in the centre or the team. There are lots of chiefs, and how well the indians get on together depends to a great extent on how well the chiefs get on with each other.

In many ways, things would be much easier if there *was* a single boss. There are many GPs who think this, and who naturally consider themselves to be the automatic choice for the role. There are many health administrators who take a similar view—similar, that is, in all respects but one. Rather than have the doctors running the show, they would be happy if the GPs were placed firmly under the control of the health authority, so that they themselves could call the tune. But, as yet, there is no sign of authority being concentrated in anybody's hands, and the situation has to be dealt with as it is. Some GPs have set up their own multi-practice medical centres, and employ their own receptionists and secretaries, centre manager, and practice nurses. A few have even thought about trying to employ their very own social worker. But they still have to work with people employed by the health authority and social services and in no way can they be said to be absolute masters of everything that goes on in their own building. They still face the kind of problems which doctors employed in health authority built centres have to contend with.

At first sight, the idea of an integrated team seems quite incompatible with having different members being responsible to different people, and having no single, mutually recognised leader. Failure to develop an effective primary health care team is often blamed on the fact that so many diverse individuals insist on inserting their own oar. The GP members argue that all would have been well if they had been allowed to take charge; senior nursing officers complain that the doctors are unwilling to compromise and always insist on having their own way. Primary health care teams and health centres are meant to bring together the several sectors involved in the delivery of primary health care, but there are plenty of people who feel that effective teams and health centres cannot develop as long as there remain divisions between these sectors at other levels. They ask how there can be integration on the ground where the work gets done, if real divisions persist at higher levels. It is a fair question. Some of the general practitioners most enthusiastic about a team approach feel that a proper team can only be achieved if they are allowed to get on with the job of creating one, free from what they consider to be unnecessary restrictions imposed by health authorities and departments of social services. Many doctors distinguish between 'full' members of the team (under their own authority) and people who only partly belong, because they are responsible to others. Nurses and health visitors often complain that they are not fully accepted as team members but add that they do not see themselves as full members anyway, for, after all, they remain responsible to their own superiors not to the GPs.

There are many kinds of team, however, and those who do not see how a primary health care team can exist the way things are at present are really thinking in terms of the wrong model. The primary health care team can, and probably should, develop with no single overall leader, and with its members responsible to different individuals and bodies. In this way, each member gets the fullest opportunity to play his or her own part, and gives the other members and the patients the fullest benefit of his or her own expertise. No one achieves overall dominance, and insists on giving the orders even in situations where others might know best. The primary health care team has to be a team of equals, or there really is no point in its existing at all. If it is run on authoritarian lines, much of the skill and knowledge that it contains is going to be wasted.

Having different members of the team responsible to different people does avoid the risk of one individual taking over completely, but it poses problems too. Team members can only work together well if those who exercise authority over them also work well together. Integration at ground level requires integration at higher levels. When senior officers are in dispute with each other their minions have a habit of becoming pawns in their squabble, and consequently have no hope of being allowed to develop any kind of close working relationship.

This does not only apply to the practice team itself, of course. It applies to the whole health centre. Because the majority of people who work in a centre are not free agents their actions are going to be, at least in part, dependent on what their superiors want them to do. The correlation between their actions and the wishes of their superiors may not always be as great as the latter might wish, but nonetheless it is bound to exist to some extent.

Quite a lot of responsibility for the success of the health centre, and for the success of its individual primary health care teams, therefore rests upon the shoulders of everyone who is in a position to exercise authority over someone in the health centre or team. People cannot be *compelled* to work together closely and effectively, and the various superiors cannot produce total harmony and liaison simply by passing down orders to that effect. But if all those in authority ensure that they are all in reasonable agreement about what they want and how they want things done, they have at least some chance of encouraging decent integration among their subordinates. If the bosses are in discord and disarray, there is little prospect for anything better among the bossed.

The GP occupies a peculiar position in at least one respect: he is usually the only one in the health centre and in the team who is more or less his *own* boss. He may well be an employer in his own right of reception and secretarial staff, and perhaps of practice nurses. He may well resent the fact that he is not in sole charge of everyone he works with. His relationship with people in the team and centre who do not come under his authority is very much dependent upon the nature of his relationship with those who *do* exercise authority over them. All too often there is conflict here instead of co-operation, and this does nothing for the chances of an *effective* primary health care team developing, or for the prospect of proper teamwork in the health centre as a whole. Frequently, the GP has to be convinced that progress is not dependent upon his elevation to divinity: good things can still happen even if he is not himself allowed to play god over everyone he works alongside. He has to be shown that he is wrong in believing that if there is more than one cook in the kitchen, they will not get around to switching on the gas, let alone spoiling the broth. He has to be shown this by practical demonstration.

It has to be made clear to the GP that nursing officers, senior social workers, and so on, have something valuable to contribute to the development of his working relationships with their subordinates, and that they do not simply get in the way. Ideally, there should be mutual understanding, goodwill, and good communications between the GP and all the relevant superiors. When the exact opposite of this applies, and where no-one sees why it should be up to him (or her) to make the first friendly move, things can go very badly.

Dr Carter was a large and energetic man, the comparatively young senior partner of a group of four. He had definite ideas about most things, and he had very definite ideas about the kind of practice team he wanted. Coming into the health centre had been all his own idea. Nobody else had been particulary bothered either way, or, if they had been against it, they had not felt inclined to say so. As far as everyone was concerned—partners or receptionists—he was a dictatorial figure. He thought that he was a benevolent dictator, but the others were not quite so sure.

He employed a veritable army of receptionists and secretaries, and there was never any question that they should be 'taken over' by the health authority when they moved into the centre. He also had three practice nurses who worked entirely in the treatment room. There were, in addition, a health authority nurse, a midwife, and two health visitors attached to the practice, and it was they who were the focus of his discontent. He started off by behaving as if he was paying their wages too and no-one else had any say in the matter of what they did. To begin with the nurse, the midwife, and the health visitors did not seem to

84

mind. So he had them doing all kinds of things that they were not supposed to do. Eventually, of course, the various officers concerned came to hear of what was going on, and they put a stop to all his innovations. They did not say anything directly to Dr Carter, they just had words with their respective subordinates, leaving them with the unfortunate task of telling him that things had changed. He was naturally furious, and some of his fury fell upon them, which they did not consider to be particularly fair. He spent much of the next few days making abusive telephone calls and writing threatening letters to the nursing officers, but the opposition seemed fully equal to him. Over the next few months he tried on several occasions to introduce some new idea. But never successfully. If he was not actually engaged in a disagreement, he was contemplating the next battle, or thinking about the last one. And this coloured his attitude towards everyone in the health centre who happened to be connected with the health authority. As far as he was concerned, you were either for him or your were against him. The population of the health centre being what it was, he was convinced that most people in the building were in fact against him, and he developed quite a complex about it. He dearly wished that he was back in his old premises.

Disagreement between GPs and people in authority is most likely where the former are, in fact, progressive in their ideas and anxious to develop real team relationships. They will have their own ideas on what contribution the nurse, health visitor, or social worker could make to the practice team, and inevitably these will sometimes conflict with what those responsible for these people will consider practicable or reasonable. Sometimes senior officers will see themselves as defending their charges against excessive demands from the GP. Sometimes the GP will feel that he has established a good relationship with other team members, that they are quite capable of deciding among themselves precisely who should do what, and that the officers only interfere and place unnecessary restrictions on their work together. The very idea of the primary health care team involves the doctor treating those who are attached to his practice as equals, and allowing them a full say in the organisation and operation of the team; but it is difficult for him to do this if nursing officers and such like make it abundantly clear that they are not going to treat their subordinates as equals, and appear to be imposing arbitrary and unreasonable decisions upon them.

Absence of conflict is not always a cause for satisfaction. Doctors are perhaps least likely to find themselves at odds with senior nursing officers, etc. when they recognise an absolute division between their own practice and the health authority, and have no wish to bridge the gap. A GP who does not want to work at all closely with his attached nurse and health visitor will have no objection to their own superiors deciding precisely what their role should be. If he has no commitment to the concept of the primary health care team, he will consider all decisions relating to them to be entirely outside his concern. The superiors concerned may be quite happy with this; pleased that he does not try to interfere; grateful for a quiet life. But if they want their subordinates to have a better working relationship with the GP they cannot be satisfied with the quiet life. They have to involve the GP in decisions they make which involve people attached to his practice, even if this is rather like playing with fire. They have to prod the GP into discussing matters affecting the nurse, health visitor or midwife, and they have to accept the risk that he will end up arguing with them. There is no harm in a little disagreement anyway. It is often necessary if there is to be any progress at all. What has to be avoided are the kind of all-out hostilities illustrated above.

In practice it is not always easy to do this. If people are determined to fight each other, there is very little that anyone can do about it. Sometimes GPs are so hostile towards the health authority and health authority officers so antagonistic towards GPs, that disagreement between them is inevitable. But things are not always as bad as this, which is fortunate. Disagreements often start, and escalate, as a result of a simple lack of thought, and a failure to observe some pretty common-sensical rules. As with many other things, much depends upon communication.

If the doctor and the officer concerned are going to trust each other, neither can afford to act—or to appear to act—behind the other's back. A nursing officer cannot expect the GP to co-operate with her, or to accept the attached nurse as a full member of the team, if she does not keep him informed about any changes she is considering in the work of that nurse, and if she is not prepared to discuss them with him. Telling the GP nothing, and allowing him to find out only when the attached nurse is actually working in accordance with a new directive, is just plain stupid. On the other hand, so is the GP's trying to persuade the nurse or health visitor to perform some new task without first consulting the appropriate supervisor. Attempts at deliberate concealment can rarely succeed, and when the discovery is made, the nursing officer might be forgiven for vetoing the change simply because she had not been asked about it, even if she has no objection to it in its own right. Apart from this, it puts the individual health visitor or nurse in an extremely invidious position, at the end of the day she will find herself distrusted by her own superiors, and resenting the GP for his lack of consideration towards her.

There may be times when it is tempting to try to introduce some innovation unilaterally, keeping it quiet until the other side suddenly finds itself presented with a fait accompli. If opposition is anticipated, it may seem the most logical course. But it destroys goodwill, and goodwill is all important. Temporary victory may be obtained at the cost of eventual, and permanent defeat. Each side can only get its own way in any lasting sense by the agreement of the other, and there is no point in the GP, for example, trying to railroad the health authority into accepting one of his ideas if he destroys the willingness of the officers concerned to co-operate with him in future.

It may seem simplistic and naive to suggest it, but it is nevertheless largely true: frankness and openness really *is* the best policy. Throwing an idea into the arena for debate, instead of trying to get it implemented surreptitiously may not guarantee its success, of course. The opposition may be too strong for it. In any system that comes close to being democratic, everyone has to accept that he will not always get his own way. But the advantages of democracy are as real in this context as they are elsewhere. Argument may even be likely, but there is much less risk of total unreasoning conflict.

'That bloody woman', said Dr Mason,' has been in here again. Eunice (a receptionist) saw her.'

'Any idea what she wanted?' asked his partner.

'Another meeting with the nurses. I don't know what it was about. But this time I'm going to find out.'

He never did find out, however. At least, not from Miss Garside.

Miss Garside, who was the senior nursing officer, came into the health centre on average about once a month. The nurses and health visitors would be called together in preparation for her arrival, and she would remain with them for at least half an hour. She never told the doctors why she had come, or what she had said, and at first they did not mind. But as time went on they began to find the visits more and more annoying.

Things tended to happen after these meetings. Nurses and health visitors might stop doing things they had been doing for some time—like filling in forms on the doctor's behalf, or undertaking certain kinds of medical procedures. the treatment room nurse might restrict the range of services she offered.

Of course, the doctors could have found out about these changes in advance, by asking the nurses with whom they worked what Miss Garside had said. But in fact they did not, because they felt that it would be beneath their dignity to do so. They considered that they were entitled to be told by the lady herself. She obviously did not. And the more she persisted in this attitude, the more hostile towards her the GPs became.

It was not only their feelings towards Miss Garside that changed. They began to take the attached nurses and health visitors less seriously. They told them less, they involved them less in the work of the practice, because they were obviously not part of a team at all. They were subject at all times to secret orders from the health authority. What was even worse, however, was the change which occurred in the doctors' feelings towards the health centre.

By behaving as she did, Miss Garside made it clear that the health centre was essentially a health authority building—or at least had a distinct health authority 'half'— which she could enter or leave as she wished without having to inform anyone. She demonstrated that whatever might have been said about the health centre—about it creating a new era in co-operation between GPs and health authority—the divisions were just as real as they had ever been. And the doctors behaved accordingly.

If the senior nursing officer comes into the health centre, has a meeting with the nurses based in it, and then leaves without any explanation to the GPs, the latter may be excused for thinking that she is up to no good. They may go on the defensive, and become less than frank themselves, for fear of giving anything away. So the thing goes on: from bad to worse to worse. The reason for her coming may in fact have been quite honourable, but unless she makes that clear, the consequences can be the same as if it was not. People act on the basis of what they *believe* to be true, not on the basis of a truth they know nothing about. The senior nursing officer—or anyone else in comparable position—has to make a deliberate effort to acquaint the doctors with what she has been saying to the nurses who work with them. Lack of time is really no excuse at all, nor for that matter is apparent indifference among the doctors. If they do not care what she has been up to, this is something she ought to be worried about. It indicates that they are not as enthusiastic about the primary health care team as they might be, and this should give her cause for concern. So she should tell them anyway, whether they want her to or not.

Where the doctors are keen to make the most of the attachment of nurse, midwife, or health visitor, there are bound to be times when they try to move too fast, and find themselves bumping up against health authority officers seeming like prune-faced chaperones. If aunty simply says no, without explaining why, frustration is bound to breed resentment. But if she tries to give proper justification for her interference, she may at least dull the edge of the doctor's disappointment.

Decisions should not appear to be arbitrary, nor should changes in attachments. If holidays, or sickness make it essential for the nursing officer to take someone temporarily away from the practice team, she should make sure that the doctor knows about this in advance, and that he understands the reason why. Failure to ensure this will only mean that the GP is persuaded that there are indeed two sides, and that any alliance at practice level is largely a pretence, something to which the health authority is not genuinely committed and which it is happy to interfere with whenever it feels so inclined.

An outbreak of 'flu or holidays created many problems for the nursing officers of a large town in the North-East. Finding enough health visitors or nurses to do all the things that had to be done could become an almost impossible task. Working out the best possible re-allocation of personnel or combination of duties might have taxed the brain of a fair-sized computer. No wonder the ladies would look haggard on occasion. One can sympathise with them a great deal. One can understand them never getting around to informing the GPs concerned of the changes which were having to be made. Unfortunately, the GPs themselves never could understand it.

They took the view that health authority personnel are—by definition—grossly under-employed, and therefore could never reasonably use the excuse of lack of time for failing to do anything. If they were not informing the doctors of what they had decided, this could only be because they had deliberately agreed not to do so.

Many of these GPs would telephone the nursing officers and complain bitterly when they discovered that 'their own' nurse or health visitor had been replaced—albeit for only a few days—by part of a stranger. Those who complained most bitterly sometimes had the normal attachments restored for them, and this made things even worse for everyone else.

The complaints only served to convince the nursing officers that the GPs in the town were unreasonable and over-demanding, and this made them even less inclined to communicate with them. One or two of the doctors were indeed unreasonable, and probably would not have been satisfied, whatever had been done. But most would have responded sympathetically if they had been kept properly informed. If they had been made aware of the size of the problem, they would have appreciated that sacrifices had to be made. Things could have been sorted out quite amicably. Instead, conflict simply bred further conflict.

Paradoxically, the more the nursing officer interferes in the working of the primary health care team, the more she can demonstrate her value to the team members (including the GP)—providing that she goes about it in the right way. In many ways she has to accept responsibility for the development of the team. Having arranged attachments, she has to ensure that they are working well, and she has to be prepared to discuss ways in which the nurses in her charge might be more effectively used. She has to be a source of ideas herself, not just an immovable obstruction to the doctors' moments of inspiration.

At the same time she must ensure that her particular subordinates are integrating well in the health centre as a whole. She may have to encourage them to be less insular; she may also have to defend their interests. If necessary, she must use her (frequently substantial) weight to ensure that they are allowed their full say in the management of the centre, just as she previously ensured that they could play a full part in its planning.

The indians cannot co-ordinate their activities if the chiefs are not in agreement. It is important for the primary health care team and for the health centre that all who are in a position of authority are open with each other, liaise with each other, and share the same overall idea of what they are trying to achieve. In this way, but only in this way, will things be better than if they were not there at all.

Separation of authority can, if not properly handled, make it difficult for the GP to work as closely as he might with the nurse, midwife, or health visitor, but it rarely makes any kind of relationship impossible. Most GPs take the view that they naturally belong alongside these three stalwarts of the community health scene. But regarding the social worker, things are usually different. There must be very few health centres in which social workers are fully accepted, or in which they are happy to find themselves. More common are centres which opened with a visiting, or even resident, social worker, but rapidly found that they could do without her. Where social workers are still to be found in the building, they are frequently the most isolated of all, ignored and possibly abused by the GPs, and hostile towards the latter in their turn. Suggestions that they should be fully integrated members of the primary health care team are invariably ridiculed by all sides.

Accommodation for social workers was initially provided in a large health centre built in the North-West of England. A comparatively large room was provided, and was used as an office by almost all the social workers based in that town. The potential for an improvement in relationships between them and the GPs in the centre was enormous.

*The doctors could actually meet and get to know the social workers
personally. Requests to see a patient (or client) and the consequent
feedback of information could be made face-to-face. But two years after
the centre was opened, the social workers moved to another office in
another part of the town. They did not come into the health centre
again, and the doctors did not miss them.*

*During the two years in which they had shared the same building,
neither the GPs nor the social workers had done anything to improve
their contact with each other, or their understanding of each other.
They had, in fact, done their best to avoid each other. The social
workers regarded the doctors with suspicion and contempt, and the
feeling was definitely mutual. These attitudes had developed long before
the health centre came into existence, and no-one made the effort to
change them.*

*One of the doctors in the centre was an important figure in national
medical affairs, but rather than taking a lead to promote a better
relationship, he hated social workers with an intensity bordering on the
fanatical. He could not bear to look upon a social worker, let alone talk
to one.*

*No GP ever entered the social workers' room, and no social worker ever
crossed the floor of the centre to reach the GPs' consulting rooms.
When the Department of Social Services found itself that other office,
the relief all round was considerable.*

More than anything else, the case of the social worker has
made it clear that simply putting people into the same building
does not automatically produce an improvement in their working relationships with each other. Many other factors exert their
effect. There are GPs who, because of personal ideology or from
bitter experience, are convinced that social workers have no
worthwhile contribution to make to primary health care. But
there are other doctors who are convinced of their worth, and
would dearly love to work more closely with them. Probably
most other members of the practice team share this positive
attitude: the health visitor, the midwife, and the home nurse are
usually aware of the contribution that the social worker can
make. So if there are some practices where they would probably
never be welcome, there are others where they would be
accepted with open arms. Why then, have health centres not

produced more progress in this respect? Why must the social worker remain essentially outside the primary health care team? The answer is that integration cannot come at this level until there is a marked narrowing of the great divide at the administrative heights. Until this happens, it is a waste of space and money allocating rooms to social services in health centres.

Because of the manner of their organisation, particular social workers are rarely associated with particular health centres or particular practice teams. It is more usual for several social workers to be involved with the patient population of one centre, and for each of those workers to have case-loads which cover the patients of other practices and centres too. There is no one-to-one involvement; no opportunity for individual social workers to identify with practice team and health centre, or to be so identified.

The health centre described here is dismally typical of many. No social workers were housed within it, and the relationship between social workers and GPs, health visitors, nurses and midwives hardly existed. By no means all the doctors in the centre recognised a need for social workers, or for any kind of involvement with them. But some did, and they regretted how bad things were.

Because there was no one-to-one relationship between practice and social worker, it was impossible to know which social worker might deal with a particular patient. Because the social workers and the members of the practice team did not know each other personally, there was no sense of mutual responsibility. Neither side cared about the other. Neither side felt an obligation to feed back information, and consequently feedback was invariably inadequate and frequently non-existent. Patients (clients) were sometimes given conflicting advice or information.

Some GPs tried to use health visitors to do the work of the social worker. Where they agreed to this, and when their superiors did not find out about it, health visitors had to let their proper work suffer in order to engage in activities for which they were not properly trained.

Each side had its stock of tales about the other. One in particular was frequently told within the health centre. A doctor had a patient who was clearly in need of psychiatric help, but not so ill that this could be imposed upon him against his will. For several weeks, therefore, the GP tried to persuade him to become a voluntary hospital in-patient. He was finally approaching success when a well-meaning neighbour notified the local social services department to see if they could do something about the poor conditions in which the man was living. A social worker duly went along, knowing nothing of the man's medical history or the preceding efforts of the GP. As a result, the effect of those efforts was entirely dissipated, and several more months went by before the patient agreed to receive proper treatment. Of course, each time this tale was told, it gained something by way of content or emphasis.

There may be good reasons why social workers should be organised as they are, but the concern here is with how health centres can be used to promote better working relationships, and consequently it must be said that unless particular social workers are allocated to particular health centres and work exclusively with the health centre practice teams, it is a waste of time having social workers in such buildings at 'all. There is no value in providing office space within the health centre if the social workers who use it have no other attachment to the centre.

There are many social workers, of course, who are absolutely opposed to their being attached to GPs' patient lists. They fear that this would somehow damage their own professional status, and indicate their subservience to the doctor. Maybe they are right. But in larger health centres, it cannot do them any harm to work in a small, permanent group exclusively serving that centre's patient population.

When one of the largest health centres in the country was being planned, the doctors decided amongst themselves that they would only have social workers in the building if they were formally attached to the individual practices. The social workers would have none of it. But there was enough goodwill and good sense on both sides to ensure that a compromise was reached. The compromise was, that a group of social workers would be based in the health centre to deal only with health centre patients.

When the health centre opened with this arrangement in operation, the progress achieved was further capitalised upon. Some GPs and some social workers realised that even more would have to be done if a substantial improvement in relationships between social services and the practice teams was to be achieved. The well-established negative stereotypes would have to be shown to be false. People would have to be given the opportunity to get to know each other, appreciate each other's skills, and, most of all, develop a mutual trust.

Joint meetings on subjects of common interest—drug addiction, abortion, alcoholism—were therefore arranged, and people who were not initially inclined to attend were persuaded by their colleagues to do so. The consequences of this initiative were quickly seen. Apart from being useful in their own right, the meetings had a positive effect on liaison between social workers and GPs, health visitors, nurses and midwives. At least some of the patients benefited greatly. So too did the health visitors, who could now get on with their own work without having to worry about sorting out social problems.

Not all GPs changed their attitudes or their way of working. It would have been unreasonable to expect this. There are still some who cannot—or will not—see the value of any kind of working contact with social workers. But given time, and enough sustained effort, they may do so yet.

Things to do with Girls

The distribution of authority, as it affects health centres, is largely a permanent and unchangeable thing. The nurses and the social workers have their respective hierarchies, and even if the GP does disapprove of them, there is nothing he can do to change them. However, there is one important group of people about whom a decision does have to be made, and who frequently find that moving into a health centre means working for a different boss. These are the receptionists and secretaries who hitherto were employed by the GPs.

Doctors contemplating a move to health centre premises have to ask themselves the question: 'What do we do with the girls?' They can, among other things, continue to pay their wages themselves, or they can ask the health authority to take them over. And if the health authority does take them on, it then has to decide whether it will allow them to continue working more or less as before, 'attached' to their original practices, or whether it will place them in a common pool.

Each of these solutions has its own advantages and disadvantages. They have all been adopted in some health centres, and adopted for different reasons. They each have different implications for the job-satisfaction of the receptionists, for the working of the primary health care team, and for integration of the health centre as a whole.

When the doctors decide to leave things as they are, this is usually because they recognise just how important the reception and secretarial staff are to the well-being of the practice team. They realise that they play an important part in the communications between other team members, and that their commitment to the team is indispensable if it is to be able to function smoothly and effectively. Furthermore, they believe that if the receptionists were to be taken on to the health authority's payroll, their loyalty to the doctors particularly would suffer, and they would be less conscientious in their work. Some GPs rather cynically argue that health authority employees are not expected to work very hard, and that the receptionists' contribution to the practice would decline somewhat if they were allowed to join their ranks. By retaining control of the whip themselves, they can ensure that the last ounce of effort continues to be extracted from them.

There are some GPs who have no strong feelings either way, but who accede to the wish of the receptionists themselves to remain in the doctors' employ. These receptionists are invariably happy with their existing relationships with the doctors, consider them to be understanding and considerate employers, and feel that the health authority would be an impersonal and inflexible boss.

What are the consequences of receptionists and secretaries continuing to work for the GPs? The advantages are undoubtedly very important ones. First of all, the receptionists tend to have high job-satisfaction, particularly where each practice has its own reception area. They retain a sense of involvement with the team, and have the gratification of knowing that they are still considered to be a necessary part of it. As a result, they are more inclined to make extra effort, and to help team colleagues beyond the call of normal duty—the occasions when the doctor has to get out the whip are mercifully rare.

Secondly, a great deal of good is done to the maintenance of practice identity in the health centre. The patients are dealt with by the same receptionists they knew in the old premises, and therefore immediately realise that the practice still exists as an autonomous unit, and has not simply become part of a larger whole. In addition, there is no disruption of the working of the team as a result of 'strange' receptionists being assigned to it. To do her job effectively, the receptionist has to get to know all the idiosyncrasies of her colleagues, or at least all of those which have any relevance to what they get up to during the working day. An appreciation of those idiosyncrasies does not only save herself time and effort, it allows her to save the time and effort of other people too. If she is replaced by someone who does not know the 'little ways' of team members, it is surprising just how difficult things can become, and just how long they can take. Besides which, a failure to satisfy the petty whims of doctor, nurse, or health visitor, can cause them to become annoyed, and this disrupts things even further. It is hard to credit just how furious some people can become if their coffee does not arrive at exactly the right time, or if their mail is opened when it should not be, or is not opened when it should.

The disadvantages of GPs continuing to employ their own receptionists in the health centre are precisely the advantages of the other systems.

If the health authority becomes responsible for all reception and secretarial staff in the health centre, and if it decides not to divest itself of the services of at least some of the doctors' original staff (as it may well do), it then has to decide whether it should allow all the ladies to work in conjunction with the practices by which they were previously employed. Quite a number of GPs and receptionists consider this to be the ideal solution. The working of the team is not necessarily disrupted, and doctors and receptionists get the benefit of the latter having a new boss. For the doctors, this benefit is mainly relief from the onerous tasks of administration which fall upon any employer. Another solution to this problem is available, however, for those who prefer it. A practice manager, or someone who plays the part without necessarily being glorified by the name, can take over these tasks and leave the doctor free for other things.

Where receptionists themselves anticipate advantages from being taken over by the health authority, the benefits they anticipate are usually financial. It is frequently believed that the health authority will pay more than the doctors, and it is probably often true. Where the doctors continue to pay their own staff in the health centre, discrepancies between what they pay and what the health authority pays comparable staff in the centre, may well lead to dissatisfaction and pressure for a wage increase. At least one group of GPs have found themselves with a strike on their hands for this reason.

The health authority often feels this system to have another advantage, which is presumably not recognised as such by the receptionists. This is that placing all receptionists and secretaries under a single employer will somehow increase their efficiency, and eventually lead to a need for fewer staff. This may be true, although there does not seem to be any real evidence to support it. It certainly does not square with the doctors' view of an overstaffed and inefficient health administration—but some will say that the GPs are prejudiced.

The main advantage of the scheme from the point of view of the working of the practice team is that although continuity of receptionists is maintained, at holiday times or during periods of sickness it is usually an easy matter to arrange for reception-ists who normally work with other practices to help out. Where the doctors are the employers even when all the practices in the health centre share a common reception area, each practice usually has to muddle through on its own when temporarily short-staffed.

The disadvantages of health authority employment of recep-tionists even when they continue to work with their original practice teams, are usually subtle, but significant. The reception-ists frequently complain that their relationship with the GPs has changed for the worse. They may find it hard to be specific, but are prone to insist that things are not as 'friendly' as they were, that the doctors do not take the same interest in them person-ally, and that they do not feel the same loyalty to the doctors in turn. Maybe this is a feeling that the GPs can remove, with a bit of effort, but if it has no basis in fact and is purely a result of their handing over responsibility for the receptionists to others,

98

there is not very much they can do about it. Certainly some ladies feel that is is somewhat ungracious of the GPs to unload them when they have worked for them for several years, and always—as they see it—done a good job.

The receptionists may see what the GPs have done as an act of betrayal, and an act of rejection. Some are fond of describing their relationship with the GPs in family terms, and if they are disposed of, might feel the hurt keenly. This has consequences for their day-to-day work in the health centre. The receptionist may still be attached to the same practice, but if she no longer feels the same commitment to it, if she is no longer quite so happy in her work, she will make the team suffer as a result. She might not be deliberately difficult—although she could be—but she will certainly not be prepared to put in any unnecessary effort, or to do more than she is paid to do.

All this can be true even when—before they actually moved into the centre—the receptionists were generally in favour of becoming health authority employees, and looking forward to the extra cash. The grass has a habit of looking greener on the other side, and when the change has been made, the reception-ists may exaggerate just how pally things were in the past. They may remember the doctors as being friendlier than they ever were in reality, but the present will seem all the worse in comparison, and their reaction will be all the greater.

If the health authority does employ the reception and secretar-ial staff itself, it has the choice of throwing them unceremoni-ously into a common pool, and pulling them out to do any job it thinks fit, regardless of their previous allegiances. It may adopt a scheme of 'rotation', so that each lady does a different job each week, and consequently becomes familiar with all the various reception roles in the health centre. This system has its own particular advantages, but its disadvantages should be obvious.

In one health centre in which this system was tried, it appeared to be working well. Because she got to know every reception role, each receptionist could take on any job when called on to provide cover at holiday times, or when someone was ill. Serious disruption to the work of each practice team and the health centre as a whole was thereby minimised. The receptionists even reported greater job-satisfaction because, they said, their work was much more varied than it used to be.

99

But perhaps this advantage was over-stated, since, in reality, the variation could not be all that great. The real cost of this solution was what it did to the primary health care teams.

Maybe it was felt that in a health centre accommodating only three separate practices, it would be possible for the receptionists to get to know everyone well, and to be able to work effectively with each practice team. In practice, they were prevented from becoming equally loyal and committed to each of them because the teams were themselves a long way from being integrated with each other, and because relationships across the health centre as a whole were not particularly good. If this extreme degree of integration had existed, they might have had some hope of serving everybody well. As it was, they each had their own favourites, and how well they worked depended on which particular practice they happened to be working for at the time.

The fact that each group of doctors had a different receptionist responsible for making appointments and handling its patients each week, caused a fair amount of confusion in the minds of those patients. Older people particularly—who were regular visitors to the health centre—were often unhappy that they could no longer deal with and get to know a single individual. They had once relied considerably upon the receptionist for explanation and reassurance. Now they could do so to a lesser extent. They had no friend between themselves and the doctor, and the GP consequently seemed a more distant and forbidding figure. These unfortunate patients might be forgiven for thinking what one of their number said: 'I liked it better when the doctors had their own place. Everything was much simpler then.'

The balance of benefit must lie with GPs hanging onto their own receptionists. This is definitely best for the primary health care team, and because promoting the team is the primary goal, the alternative benefits conferred by alternative schemes must be considered less significant. If the health authority takes them on instead, even more chiefs are introduced as far as the team and the health centre are concerned. The receptionists will have new superiors, and what the receptionists do will depend on them. If the GPs do voluntarily give up direct control of their own reception and secretarial staff, they should have some pretty firm guarantees that the new bosses will work with them, not against them or independently of them. Whoever is given responsibility for the receptionists must liaise closely with the GPs and other team workers, because if they do not they can do the practice teams concerned a great deal of harm. The receptionist is a key figure in any health centre, and a vital member of the team—she has to be treated as such. She particularly has to be treated as such when she has to be replaced. And the GP, as well as everyone else in the team, has to be consulted when new appointments are made. But this is a subject for the next chapter.

CHAPTER SIX

The Matter of Personalities

Choosing the Company

Compared with many things in this life, breeding mice is easy. You get enough of each sort, put them all in the same cage, and wait. You do not even have to wait very long. Perhaps you could say that mice are promiscuous; you might also say that they are single-minded. The only thing they consider is gender. Beyond that, they do not seem to have any preferences.

Now what happens if you pick up some doctors, nurses, health visitors, and receptionists, and anyone else who seems appropriate, and drop *them* down together in their very own health centre cage? It could be anything; and exactly what does happen depends on a great many things, like what they think of each other for instance.

Feelings can change, of course, and because we are very much influenced by our surroundings, such change can often be attributed to environmental factors. Some situations are much more romantic than others. A health centre can provide a setting that encourages its participants to adopt a more positive attitude towards each other by having its counterparts of moon, martinis, and Mediterranean. No one can be blamed for failing to get excited in a centre reminiscent of a wet weekend in Seaton Sluice. Health centres are supposed to promote amicability and mutual respect in place of suspicion, ignorance and a sense of opposing sides, and if they are properly made they can go a long way towards achieving this. But sometimes feelings are so strong that nothing will change them. Whatever environment they find themselves in, some people will never get on together. If they happen to find themselves sharing the same health centre, the centre itself—however excellent a place it might be—will not change them. Their mutual antagonism will survive intact, and it is the health centre which will suffer. The more incompatible are the individuals who populate it, the greater is the centre's failure going to be as far as its goal of promoting better working relationships is concerned. All the other efforts will have been in vain if the people who eventually move into the new premises are so opposed in terms of personalities or objectives that they will, at best, avoid each other, and at worst engage in open conflict. The centre will have no hope of success. A good health centre can only do its stuff if it is given a chance.

Importing long-standing feuds into brand new health centres is tantamount to sabotage. A health centre is supposed to be a place where people with diverse skills in primary health care can work together, not a field of battle or an arena for gladiatorial contest. So it would seem an obvious point that people who are known to be antagonistic towards each other should not be encouraged to practice from the same building. But there are centres where participating group practices were known to have disliked each other for donkey's years, and where the administrator largely responsible would seem to have arranged this on purpose so that he might be able to enjoy the spectacle of two lots of doctors fighting it out.

If you were so inclined, you might in fact assume that anyone who encourages mutually antagonistic groups to move into the same building must either be short on brains or have a perverted and sadistic sense of fun. But there is another, and, perhaps, kinder explanation. It relates to this assumption that building health centres is what matters, not building *successful* health centres, or health centres that really provide value for money. There are health administrators whose first aim is to get GPs into health centre premises. The more GPs they can get into such premises the better.

There was once a Medical Officer of Health who had dedicated himself to this end. He was determined that every part of his—quite extensive—domain should have a health centre in it, and once a particular scheme had been launched, he devoted great energy to ensuring that the largest possible number of GPs should become involved with it. Much work was done 'behind the scenes' to convince all who had doubts, of the benefits of health centre practice. But the favourite technique was the organised meeting.

Representatives of all the practices in the area would be invited to attend, and encouraged to do so by the promise of free food and drink. The project would then be 'sold' to the audience with considerable skill and numerous illustrations, and when this was completed the MoH would sit at a table with a large sheet of paper before him, and his fountain pen in his hand.

'Now, gentlemen', he would say. 'Who can we count on?'

Some, of course, had already decided to come into this centre. Others were uncertain, but became intoxicated by the occasion, and gradually the list of intending participants grew longer. The longer it grew, the more pressure the uncommitted felt upon themselves to go in with the rest; and the longer it grew, the more delighted the MoH was seen to be. As things narrowed down to the last few resisters, the atmosphere within the room became electric. The red-faced MoH would mop his brow, and the pen would shake in his hand. And if, as often happened, all were eventually persuaded, he would find it impossible to contain himself, and would dance about the room, laughing uncontrollably and shaking hands with everyone in sight.

With administrators like this, anyone who shows interest will be welcomed enthusiastically, regardless of who he is, and regardless of what his reasons for showing interest might be. Anyone who does not want to work in a health centre will find himself a target for persuasion, and especially so where all the other doctors responsible for a particular area or town have decided to move into new, shared premises. When this occurs, the odd man out—the odd group out—is going to come under every possible pressure to conform with the rest. 'Getting them all in' becomes an end in itself, and failure can hardly be contemplated. Every effort would be made to prevent it. And if those efforts were successful, and the sinner grudgingly agreed to go along with the rest, there would be more rejoicing in the health authority offices than over all the other general practitioners who actually wanted to work in a health centre. There would be rejoicing simply because the last practice had been brought into the fold, and nothing else would matter. It would not matter that a long-standing quarrel had aiso been brought in. It would not matter that as a result of this success, the health centre would inevitably be crippled by argument and acrimony and would have no hope of reaching its full potential. But it ought to matter. The success of the health centre should not be sacrificed on the altar of getting as many people as possible under the one roof. If harmony and good relationships depend upon some individuals or groups being left out, then they should be left out.

Trying to ensure the compatibility of the people who form the initial working population of a health centre is not just a matter of keeping out those who have long been in disagreement. It would be easy if it were. The dispute would probably be well-known, and, anyway, the combatants would be unlikely to wish to practice in the same building. But it cannot be assumed that if disagreements have not existed in the past, they will be unlikely to emerge in the health centre. It cannot even be assumed that people will get on well together in their new, shared premises because they have got on well together previously. Hitting it off, so to speak, in one situation, does not guarantee a similar result when the circumstances are different. People who enjoy each other's company when they are housed in separate premises and are not compelled to interact may find that living under the same roof leads them to see each other in a new light, and changes the very nature of their relationship.

The old surgery of Dr Secombe and partners was but a short distance from that of Drs Porter, Carver and Burns, but, short as it was, the distance turned out to have been very necessary. On a personal basis, these two groups of doctors got on very well. They always had done. Their practices were quite independent of each other, and no-one wanted to change that, but when both began to wish for something more spacious and modern in the way of premises, it was perhaps inevitable that they should consider the possibility of sharing a health centre. The Medical Officer of Health, as he was then, was quite enthusiastic about the idea, and so—with considerably more effort and delay than might be suggested by this simple statement—a health centre was built.

In addition to the Secombe and Porter practices, it accommodated a good range of health authority services, and was opened with high hopes for its future. Certainly no-one predicted how big a disaster it would turn out to be.

Being such good friends, the two groups of doctors saw no objection to their sharing reception and waiting areas. This was perhaps fortunate, because their opinion on the matter was not asked anyway. They also shared the use of a treatment room, and the services of a treatment room nurse. This treatment room, and the nurse attached thereto, eventually became a focus of disagreement; but it was in the reception area that friendship suffered its first major attack.

It soon became clear that if the doctors were old friends, the two groups of receptionists which they employed were not. The very smallness of the area allotted to them forced them to compete for space, and more or less from the outset they resented each other's presence. After only a few days, quarrelling broke out, and innocently, with the best of intentions, Dr Secombe intervened. He addressed his kindly avuncular remarks to the 'girls' whose wages he paid, and then, confident that Sammy Porter would not mind, had a word with the combatants on the other side. Unexpectedly, Sammy Porter did mind. He reacted bitterly, and Dr Secombe was quite taken aback. He could not understand it at all.

Dr Porter was, in fact, already a little disillusioned with the health centre, and was wondering if he had not made a mistake in coming in. His initial complaint was not with the Secombe practice. It was simply that he found the presence of so many people around him somewhat oppressive. In a way he could not define, he felt that his privacy was somehow being infringed. He told his wife that it was like practising medicine in a goldfish bowl. He realised how much happier he had been in his old surgery, and the knowledge that he could not go back there—the demolition men having moved in the day he moved out—deepened his depression. The only crumb of comfort was the fact that Secombe and his partners were not proving obtrusive. They seemed equally anxious to keep to themselves. So when Dr Secombe played uncle with Sammy's receptionists, it was a case of et tu doctor, and the hurt was all the more painful for that. Dr Secombe's attempt at any explanation did not help either. It merely demonstrated to Sammy that his own receptionists were unhappy too, and that they did not enjoy having to share premises with another practice. Then the treatment room came into it.

107

Mrs Jabb, the treatment room nurse, found herself a great deal busier than she had expected to be. She said that she was not complaining about this, but she managed to give a lot of people the impression that she was. When she mentioned the matter to Dr Secombe, he certainly got the impression that she was demanding that something be done about it. He wondered if it might not be possible for the home nurses connected with the two health centre practices to help out in the treatment room at busy times of the day. The next time he saw the senior nursing officer, he mentioned this idea to her, even though he had not yet had a chance to discuss it with Dr Porter.

In the old days, Dr Porter would have been happy that his friend had taken the initiative. But now he was looking at things from a different perspective. He greatly resented Secombe making plans for 'his' nurse, and, as he saw it, sneakily trying to get them implemented behind his back.

From then on, relations between the two groups deteriorated steadily. They rarely spoke to each other, and avoided each other as much as possible. They stopped using the common room. They even began to demand that the health authority rebuild the centre—at great expense—in order to provide complete physical segregation of the one group from the other.

It might be thought that if two practices are already on good terms with each other, they would be able to cope with having to share things like waiting and reception areas. They would be unlikely to get worried about their separate identities and they would be unlikely to find each other's very close proximity significantly troublesome. But people who are compatible in one situation can be a long way from it in another. The trouble is, they very often do not realise this until it is too late. They think that because they have been happy enough with a well separated co-existence, they will be quite content with, might even enjoy, life in a building in which their respective working spaces actually overlap. It is easy for them to say this when they have not tried it, and are smilingly unaware of all the niggling implications. But surviving on amicable terms when daily contact cannot be avoided, when each is forever getting in the other's way, and when the reception area was manifestly not designed for receptionists of Mrs Nimble's elephantine proportions or of Miss Chester's degree of mammary development, calls for an amount of tolerance and goodwill that not everybody possesses. Where two or more groups of doctors who consider themselves friends contemplate moving into the same health centre, they would do well to think carefully on the question whether their friendship would survive the move. They may decide that it will, but they should at least consider the matter carefully, and take nothing for granted.

Having to share space with other practices in the health centre can often create hostility where none existed before, but even where the centre provides autonomous practice areas it is by no means inevitable that relationships which were satisfactory enough in the old days will continue that way in the new premises. Perhaps doctors in two separate groups developed a mutual liking and respect because they were very like each other in terms of interests and objectives—that similarity between them might turn out to be a veritable *cause* of disagreement when they come to share the same focus for their goals and interests. This was the case with the Strong and Keen groups.

Dr Strong liked Dr Keen. And, for that matter, Dr Keen liked Dr Strong. They had the same attitudes on a lot of things, and particularly on general practice, health authority officers, whisky and golf. They each dominated their own group, and eagerly sought to make their practices as efficient and up-to-date as they could be. They were dedicated to innovation and imposed it rigorously, tolerating no dissent from receptionist or partner alike. They demanded obedience, they demanded respect, and believed implicitly in the supreme effectiveness of a dictatorial style of government. This meant that everyone else in the Strong practice had a great deal in common with everyone else in the Keen practice: a down-trodden appearance, a strong sense of inferiority, and a highly unstable life. Consequently, they too found themselves drawn together. There were many evenings when they would meet in the pub, and indulge in mutual sympathy and ale until they reached the point where things did not seem too bad after all.

Dr Strong and Dr Keen were equally looking forward to getting into the health centre. Each was gleefully anticipating a greater scope for his energies, a greater kingdom upon which to exercise his will. And when the centre opened both went to it with a vigour unusual even for them.

109

But two kings in one kingdom is bound to lead to trouble sooner or later, and the rate at which they were moving meant that they bumped into each other very much on the sooner side. Within only a matter of days they were fighting hammer and tongs, and everyone else got so caught up in the conflict that the health centre rapidly reached that state of chaos and despair invariably found where there is civil war. Years have now gone by, and things are still the same. The only hope is that the struggle will eventually take its toll of the two combatants: that Strong will weaken, or that Keen will lose his enthusiasm. But there is no sign of that yet.

Now if some people find each other's company pleasant because they are much alike, there are some who are attracted by differences. Like can attract like, but so too—of course—can unlike. In terms of using the health centre in order to promote change, and to encourage progress in general practice, it makes a kind of sense to put dissimilar groups in the same building. A group which has not changed its style of working since the formation of the National Health Service might be prompted to bring itself up to date by the close proximity of another group dedicated to the latest way of doing things. The very existence of differences invites comparison, and suggests taking a fresh look at oneself: both sides can benefit. But, here again, there are no universal rules. People with different ideas and attitudes might not influence each other; they might simply disagree, and go on disagreeing. As happened with the health centre described back in Chapter 3, the old-fashioned group can resent the 'pushiness' and conceit of the go-ahead doctors, and the latter can look upon them in turn with contempt and annoyance, blaming them for holding the health centre back.

Some cynical individuals might suggest that there is not a pair of practice groups in the country really fit to be in the same health centre. There might even be an element of truth in the suggestion. If health centres were only to be staffed with people who could be guaranteed to work together peacefully and amicably, there would be very few centres anywhere. Common-sense has to be used—yet again—over this matter of compatibility, and it has to be recognised that it is probably always going to be one of degrees of *in*compatibility. People are rarely going to be perfect for each other, and it is the *real* incompatibilities that have to be avoided. How to avoid them, how to spot the people who are going to come to hate the sight of each other and reduce the health centre to a shambles in the wake of their conflict, cannot be the subject of universal advice. It requires knowing everyone concerned, and knowing them pretty well: knowing them well enough to decide under what circumstances old friends might become new enemies and whether quite dissimilar men, or women, might actually enjoy the experience of working closely together, and come to benefit from it.

It is important that the doctors who propose to move into a health centre should have the opportunity to find out for themselves whether or not they are going to be able to tolerate each other's constant and close presence. Some of them will doubtless know each other fairly well already, but in circumstances quite different from those that will apply in the centre. Giving everyone a trial run in health centre premises along the lines of trial marriage is unfortunately not a realistic possibility. An alternative is for all concerned to have the clearest possible idea of what life in a health centre is like by visiting centres that have been in operation for some time, and by talking to the people who work in them. As was mentioned earlier, one advantage of involving everyone in the planning process is that they will be given the opportunity of getting to know each other, and hearing each other's attitudes and intentions as they relate to the centre. If the doctors of one group do not like what they hear, they can pull out of the project before they have committed themselves too far, by disposing of their existing premises, for example.

Having a practice pull out during this stage can be a considerable nuisance to the health authority. They are faced then with the problem of finding a replacement practice, or—if this cannot be done—re-designing the centre to cater for fewer groups. But it is better, far better to have problems at this stage, than to have them emerge when the centre is actually in operation. It is better to have the problem of replacing a potentially dissident group than to have to cope with constant tensions and disagreements in an operating health centre. The administrators who take the view that they should try to get the place built with the minimum of fuss, are wrong—dangerously, and sometimes expensively, wrong. By failing to give people the opportunity to decide whether or not they are going to be happy with the communal life, they avoid difficulties for themselves before the centre is opened only at the risk of having a centre whose works are permanently clogged by the incompatibility of its participants. Ensuring a successful health centre in which all who work in it have the potential to develop better liaison and mutual understanding is not compatible with a quiet life in the days—or years—of planning and construction.

If one group of individuals conclude that their relationship with others in the proposed health centre is going to be a long way from pleasant, they are likely to change their plans. But human nature being the enigma that it is, they may not do. They may insist on coming into the centre, even though they know that they will be constantly in a state of war. And even without these entirely incompatible individuals there is inevitably going to be some degree of mis-match among people working in most health centres. Complete harmony in a health centre population has to be as rare as it is in any other form of social unit—and that means it is exceedingly rare. There are bound to be some individuals who do not think much of each other. But if incompatibilities cannot be avoided altogether, they must at least be recognised, and consequent action taken. Trouble has to be anticipated, and there has to be somebody in the health centre to deal with it when it comes: to head it off before it can gain real momentum and cause real damage. A competent and perceptive health centre manager can make a pretty good best of a fairly bad job.

Difficult as this may be for some to believe, GPs do not necessarily pose the greatest problem as far as compatibility is concerned. Because of their relatively powerful position in the health centre, a conflict involving them can cause a lot of incidental damage. But other people can be troublesome too: receptionists, for example.

During the planning stage of one health centre project, the doctors involved got to know each other better than they had done previously, and did not foresee any problems when they should all come to be based in the same building.

When things were well advanced, however, with the centre almost built, someone felt that it might be a good idea to arrange a gathering of all who would be working in the place, so that they all might get to know each other. The gathering was eventually held, and exceedingly well-attended. Every receptionist of the four practice groups came along, and among their number was Mrs Hunt.

Until that evening, no-one in the other practices had known of Mrs Hunt, or even suspected her existence. Single-handed, she had seen to the needs of a three man group for more than ten years, and it soon became obvious that she had had to work single-handed because no other woman would work with her. She had a very peculiar personality. For a lady, she was possessed of a sense of humour that might best be described as unusual, and she also had a very loud voice. That voice was heard throughout the entire evening, and wherever you happened to be standing in the room, you could not get away from it. It did not take a great deal of imagination to realise what sharing a health centre with Mrs Hunt would be like.

The next morning, a great many telephone calls were made, and the result was that the three practices newly-introduced to Mrs Hunt threatened to withdraw from the project unless the doctors who employed her got rid of her. The MoH, in desperation, asked these doctors if they would be willing to do so, but he was not surprised when they said they would not. Neither were they willing to withdraw from the health centre themselves. For a few days, disaster seemed inevitable. But then, the lady in question gave an undertaking to restrain herself in the new premises, and everyone eventually accepted this.

The health centre has now been in operation for five years and Mrs Hunt is still there. Perhaps, by her own standards she has restrained herself; and, to be fair, she has never been quite as bad as she was on that first evening. But most people do regret her presence. She is a constant source of annoyance, and the number of complaints made against her is only exceeded by the number of complaints which she herself makes about the health centre and everyone connected with it.

From time to time, the idea of a Christmas party or other social function for the health centre personnel is raised. But it never gets very far, because everyone knows that Mrs Hunt would come.

People outside the primary health care team are important too. Social workers, and people who provide health authority services are not accommodated in a health centre simply because it happens to be a convenient place to put them. At least, that *should not* be the only reason. They ought to be there because there is a desire to improve working relationships between primary health care teams, and health authority and social services. This will only happen when the doctors, nurses, health visitors and receptionists in the health centre *want* to work with them. If they do not like them as individuals, relationships will not improve, however desirable they might consider improved relationships to be in principle. The doctors and the primary health care teams constitute the core of any health centre; everyone else has to fit in with them. Some will regret it, but that is the way it is. If senior social workers genuinely want to achieve effective, practical liaison between their subordinates and practice team members, they should make every effort to ensure that the social workers they place in a health centre are likely to be able to get on reasonably well with the people who happen to be in the practice teams. This obviously applies equally to those responsible for allocating chiropodists, dentists, or anybody else of similar kind employed by the health authority. It is important to recognise that a quarrelsome individual does not only create negative relationships between himself and anyone else he is involved with. Combatants can attract sympathisers, so that eventually the whole centre is divided up into two opposing camps. It is easy enough for a disagreement between a GP and a health authority employee to remind everyone else in the centre where their true loyalty lies.

Keeping the Rockers Out

Although most of the people who come into a health centre at the outset will probably remain there for a quite considerable time, the population of any centre is unlikely to remain entirely static for very long. If new services are provided once the centre has got under way, totally new positions are going to be created; but even where this does not happen, replacements will still have to be found for those who do leave. Trying to ensure the compatibility of these replacements with everyone else is just as important as is trying to ensure the compatibility of those coming into the centre at the beginning. If a health centre is working well, and showing signs of developing along hoped for lines, it is something of a tragedy if the arrival of a newcomer causes enough disruption to set things back to where they were when the place first opened. Everybody involved with the health centre has a responsibility to endeavour to make sure that people who are obviously not going to fit in with the centre as a whole are not brought in. Unfortunately, this responsibility is rarely recognised or accepted. One of the potentially most dangerous situations arises when a practice group decides to take on a new partner.

The selection of a new doctor to join an existing practice is inevitably going to remain basically in the hands of the other doctors in the group. It is obviously unrealistic to suggest that they should allow colleagues in other health centre groups to have any say. If it is possible, they are even *less* likely to allow the involvement of any representative of the health authority or social services. But accepting this as inevitable does not mean that it is desirable that GPs should choose their new partners solely with reference to their own practice, and with total disregard for everyone else in the health centre. If a group comes into a health centre, their subsequent actions should take into account the interests of the centre. If they are unwilling to accept such responsibility and constraints, they really have no right to be in premises shared with anybody else.

Problems can arise not only when new doctors have to be found. Where the GPs continue to employ their own reception and secretarial staff, a similar situation can develop when one of their number has to be replaced. If the doctors have made a deliberate decision to continue employing their own receptionists, instead of allowing this function to be taken over by the health authority, they are likely to be much inclined to the view that who they employ is their own affair. But particularly where a shared reception area serves all the practices in the centre, it is in the doctors' own interests that they should find someone capable of working alongside the existing receptionists in comparative peace. Even if the chosen lady is well-liked by everyone in her own practice team, if she is engaged in constant dispute with her opposite numbers in other practices, her own work will inevitably suffer and the effectiveness of her own team will be reduced accordingly. A health centre manager worth his salt should therefore be able to convince the GPs of the value of seeking his advice when appointments at this level have to be made. If he goes about things the right way, having proved his worth in this, he might even be able to persuade them of the desirability of consulting him when they have to appoint one of their own status.

Where the health authority employ the receptionists, they have an opportunity to ensure that replacements are made with full consideration being given to the matter of compatibility. But, in practice, a health authority can act in as parochial a manner as any group of general practitioners. It may take the view that since it now pays the wages, and not the GPs, it has the sole right to all matters of hiring and firing. A health administrator might, quite conceivably, use the opportunity to demonstrate to the doctors that in at least one area their authority and influence had been removed. Even the health centre manager's advice need not be sought, despite his being, in all probability, a health authority employee. In fact, he might be excluded from the making of such a decision because of this: because he comes lower in the bureaucratic hierarchy than the administrator concerned, and the latter wishes to play despot.

So far, this matter of compatibility has been discussed with relation to the overall health centre population. But it is a consideration of equal importance with regard to the primary health care team itself. Ideally a new team member should be acceptable to everybody in the centre outside the team; but it should not be forgotten that he or she also has to be capable of generating satisfactory relationships with his or her own team members. There is a very strong case for saying that everyone in the team should have a voice in the selection of a new team colleague, even if it is accepted that some will inevitably be allowed to shout louder than others. It has already been said that as far as nurses, health visitors or midwives are concerned, the nursing officer responsible for making attachments should bear very much in mind the wishes of people already working in the team—and this does not mean just the doctors. Receptionists, because they play so important a role in communications within the practice team, have to be acceptable to everybody. So they have to be chosen with care, and with respect for every-body's feelings. The greatest difficulties can be created when the health authority has taken over employment of receptionists, but allows them to work in their original practice teams. The administrator concerned has to be willing to work very closely with the team if the new receptionist is to be a successful addition to it. An uncompromising health authority officer can do great damage to a primary health care team by choosing for it someone who is not going to be liked or respected by the other members. Even when the person chosen might have been acceptable in other circumstances, a high-handed attitude by the administrator, refusing to allow team members any say, is likely to provoke rejection of the recruit out of an understand-able feeling of resentment.

Keeping the Knockers Out

There is a final sense in which this question of compatibility should be considered. This is the compatibility of people with the health centre itself—with the health centre ideal, if you like. Not everyone who contemplates moving into a health centre is enthusiastic about the prospect. General practitioners move in for many reasons, and often do so *despite,* rather than because of, their feelings about health centres. Most other people have very little choice. Health authorities are generally devoted to drawing GPs into health centres, and are not very selective in consequence. They will take just about anybody who offers himself. This policy clearly cannot be very good for the goal of providing health centres which not only exist, but which also are successful and effective in providing improved primary health care. Inevitably, expensive new premises are sometimes provided for dead-beats who have not the slightest intention of putting them to good use, and ensuring that they give real value for money. Some who move into the health centre with enthusiasm are inevitably going to find their efforts sabotaged and frustrated by doctors who are entirely opposed to any kind of development of the centre, and determined to have as quiet a life as possible. Health centres cannot be restricted only to those who really believe in them. If they were, very few would be built. And a decently planned, designed, and managed health centre might expect to have some success in converting the initially lukewarm. But there are some doctors who, it is obvious right from the start, will never have any liking for the health centre, and will oppose anything that threatens to change their existing way of working. For the sake of the public who pay, for the sake of everybody else in the health centre, and for the sake of those doctors themselves, every effort should be made to persuade them not to come in. If their 'interest' in the health centre results from problems connected with their existing surgery premises—if those premises have become too costly to maintain, or are threatened with demolition—they should be helped to find another solution.

There are other people who need no persuading not to move into a health centre. They have no desire at all to make the change, and would not if they were not compelled to do so. A nurse or health visitor attached to a group of doctors who have decided in favour of the health centre will be expected to tag along with them, regardless of how she might feel about the matter. In all probability, she will be at least as keen as the GPs, and may be keener; she may have slight reservations which will quickly disappear when she has actually experienced the new premises; but she may also be unalterably opposed. Whether or not she tells the nursing officers how she feels depends on how approachable they are, and how sympathetic she feels they are likely to be. The nursing officers may not know that one of their subordinates is greatly opposed to working in a health centre, or, if they know, they may not care. Cracking the whip in such a case could be justified quite well: after all, the nurse or health visitor could only be allowed to have her way by breaking the attachment and disrupting what might be excellent team relationships. But there is a worse evil than this. If someone is forced into a health centre against his or her own will, resentment is likely to thrive, enthusiasm for the job will decline, and work will suffer. Insisting on the attachment continuing in the new premises would probably have a worse effect on the primary health care team than breaking it cleanly, and allowing a fresh start to be made with a group of people who were equally in favour of the move.

True enthusiasts are inevitably rare, and no health centre is likely to find enough of them to fill all its rooms. The best it can hope for is one or two, who might stimulate the lukewarm or indifferent majority. But this does not mean that when it comes to populating a health centre any old mob will do. Some people are bad for health centres and health centres are bad for them. An excellent primary health care team can be destroyed by a move into health centre premises, and can, at the same time, cripple the centre which has destroyed it. Some people will work happily in smaller centres, but are not fit to be in large ones. Others will feel frustrated with the limited scope of a small health centre, but will positively thrive in an enormous place offering a variety of services and with a widely qualified personnel. People are different, and to get the best from them, they have to be offered a range of situations in which to work. Health centres are not ideal for everyone. If an attempt is made to cram everyone into them, they will not succeed as they might.

CHAPTER SEVEN

Managing It

Responsibility without Power

If things are to happen in health centres, people have to make them happen. Nothing comes about automatically. It is not enough that the place is designed to encourage and facilitate the development of desired relationships. It is not enough that the building is populated by individuals who find each other's company tolerable or pleasant. It is not even enough that those individuals *want* to work more closely together. They will not succeed in doing so unless deliberate effort is made.

There are many health centres of which doctors, nurses, administrators, and various others complain that things have not developed as they wanted them to. They wonder why, and if they blame anybody, it is everybody else. None see fault in their own lack of action, in their own sitting back and waiting for developments. Maybe they will say they were waiting for someone to make the first move. Someone always has to make the first move, but individuals inclined to make it are not all that common. There *are* born leaders, of course, and with a bit of luck a health centre will have one. With a bit more luck, he (or she) will want to lead in the right direction. But neither of these fortunate occurrences can be relied upon. And anyway, a person who already has a job to do in the health centre cannot fairly be expected to shoulder the responsibility of making the centre a success. At least not on his—or her—own. The enthusiastic amateur *is* important, and should never be discouraged—after all, the ideal would be a situation in which *everyone* who worked in the centre was enthusiastic and active in promoting the centre's success. But full-time assistance is required. There has to be someone whose job it is to encourage and engineer closer working relationships among health centre participants, and to ensure that the development of health centre services is not neglected; someone who is not going to be distracted from this task by other priorities. There has to be a health centre manager. The health centre manager can help to get things going, and help to keep things going. He can help everyone who works in the centre to make the most of it, and to make the most of themselves. He cannot run the show on his own, and that is not his purpose. His role is to promote *self*-help, and his success will be measured by what others get up to: to what extent they recognise the health centre as their own, and accept responsibility for its fortunes.

The need for a health centre manager may well be disputed by many. After all, it can be said, so many health centres do not have a manager and they have not collapsed in consequence. Well, they may not have collapsed, although some have undoubtedly come close to it, but neither have they prospered as they might have done. A health centre can only be a health centre, as opposed to a building housing an unrelated and mutually disinterested collection of individuals, where it has either a manager as such, or some other over-worked and unpaid enthusiast to perform his role. Somebody has to do the organising and prod the sedentary into action. There are others who will agree that a health centre manager is well worth having, but have a very different idea of what his job should entail. According to their idea of his role, calling him a 'manager' would really be quite inappropriate. They have in mind a glorified caretaker or a glorified clerk, and maybe they would not even grant the exaltation. They might call the man who orders the toilet rolls and organises the cleaners 'health centre manager' in much the way the dustman's title has been changed in recent years to something more euphonious. But the health centre manager really has to manage. He has to be concerned with everybody in the centre, not just the ladies who scrub the floors. And this makes him a much more controversial character.

He cannot play autocrat, that goes without saying, but these days autocratic managers are not very popular anywhere. His rights and authority are strictly circumscribed, and he cannot dictate the manner in which people work together. But the manner in which they work together is his concern, and he has to guide and goad them in a positive direction with personal influence and subtle skills. He has to be the colleague of everyone in the health centre, and no way the boss, because he can only succeed with their co-operation, and the measure of his success is the degree of their co-operation—with him, and with each other. But he cannot buy co-operation at the price of leaving everyone alone. He has to make a nuisance of himself—in the nicest possible way.

Perhaps it is paradoxical, but it is in precisely those health centres where the health centre manager is least welcomed that he is most needed. If it is not paradoxical, it is at least unfortunate. Health centre managers of the kind considered here are only appointed where people concerned with the health centre are aware of its potential and keen that this should be realised. Such a centre will already have a great deal going for it. The manager's role will still be of great importance, but it will be less arduous than it might be. The need for a health centre manager is rejected and denied in those centres where the relevant administrators or participating professionals have no particular desire to see the centre really develop. The very idea of a manager is anathema to the more conservative in the field of primary health care. General practitioners jealous of their own autonomy and used to running their own affairs do not take kindly to the thought of being managed. More 'progressive' GPs are more likely to see the virtue of having such an individual, and are more likely to co-operate with him (or her). But even they may have some doubts. After all, there can be few family doctors who are *not* traditionalists at heart when it comes to the independence of their practice, and the threat of interference in their practice affairs may temper the spirits of even the most enthusiastic. The health centre manager would presumably be more amenable to all if it were made clear that his (or her) primary concern is to *safeguard* the identity and integrity of the practice team in the new premises, and not to interfere.

The manager's job is hardest in those centres where there is least commitment to the health centre ideal not only because here he has most to do, but also because he is least likely to be accepted. The health centre manager can have little authority of his own. He certainly cannot have authority over general practitioners, nor can he dictate to nursing staff or social workers or any other professional personnel. At the most, if the health authority takes over responsibility for receptionists, he may be given authority over them. Therefore, if he is going to have any beneficial effect in the health centre, he cannot achieve this by issuing directives and expecting everyone to comply whether they like it or not. He can only influence them by gaining their respect for what he has to say. Because he is not medically qualified himself, he may have something of a problem here as far as many people in the centre are concerned. He is in danger of being dismissed as a mere layman. Or worse, he may be condemned as yet another administrator by practical men and women who are not noted for their sympathy for administration. He may well have a lot of prejudice to overcome. So he has to be thick-skinned and he has to have a fair amount of self-confidence. If he suffers from something of an inferiority complex, and is on the defensive to begin with, he is not going to dare open his mouth.

Although it was decided to have a health centre manager in the Ada Ramsbottom Health Centre, built a few years ago in a certain northern town, the decision was not entirely unopposed. Some of the doctors declared the post to be unnecessary, and a reprehensible waste of money. But the MoH was very keen, and so were most of the GPs. The MoH said he had somebody in mind.

It transpired that the person he had in mind was already employed by the health authority in a clerical capacity. He was an exceedingly timid young man, who was apt to cry when offended, and who had a rather peculiar walk. In all these respects he was obnoxious to most of the people who actually worked in the centre, and even those who had favoured the appointment of a manager quickly joined in the general reaction to him. He became an object of ridicule and the butt of innumerable jokes. Being a very sensitive person, he did not take long to realise how everyone felt about him and he became greatly upset and depressed. As much as possible he hid in his office, and tried to forget about the health centre world outside his door. He seemed to feel that the only way he could become liked was to avoid doing or saying anything that anyone could possibly object to. And he was not sure just what might be objected to, so he played safe. Consequently, after a year

*had gone by and the time came for his contribution to the health centre
to be assessed, he could not recount very much that might justify his
salary. Nor did anyone else in the centre feel inclined to argue for his
retention. Having failed utterly and completely, he was promoted to a
better-paid position in the health authority hierarchy. He was not
replaced, and nobody considered that he should be.*

A health centre manager has to gain respect for himself by
showing that he is worthy of it. He has to be tactful, intelligent,
and energetic. If he can talk sensibly, show understanding, and
demonstrate his ability to get things done, he stands a good
chance of being accepted. So the health centre manager has to
have considerable qualities. This is not a job that many people
could successfully handle. And even though salary is not always
related to worth, it must be assumed that someone having the
right characteristics is going to expect reasonable remuneration.
In smaller health centres, it might be felt that there will be
insufficient work to keep such a person busy and to justify his
salary, and perhaps this will be true. It may be desirable to have
one person responsible for two or more smaller centres. It is
certainly better to have one competent and comparatively
expensive individual looking after two or three centres, than to
have relative *in*competents in each of them. A good health
centre manager can do a great deal towards making a successful
health centre; a bad manager can practically guarantee its failure
single-handed. Because his very job represents the new and
progressive, and because he is clearly identified with the health
centre itself, criticism that he deserves may be unjustly
generalised to much else that is greatly worthwhile. He can
reaffirm attitudes in those who are already unwilling to change,
and disillusion people who were originally prepared to consider
innovations in primary health care delivery. A bad choice for
this job can turn out to be a disaster.

If one person is given responsibility for more than one health
centre, gaining acceptance by all the people working in each
centre obviously becomes that bit more difficult. The manager
has to put in extra effort to demonstrate that he really is
concerned for each of his charges, and that he 'belongs' to each
centre as much as does anyone else who works in it.

Although the health centre manager may have direct

authority over no-one, someone, inevitably, will have authority over him. Usually it will be the health authority which appoints and pays him, and which will supervise his performance. But the manager cannot afford to appear to be anybody's lackey, in anybody's pocket. There will be times—perhaps there will be many times—when he has to sort out problems between the health authority and the GPs, and he cannot do this very well if he is expected to favour, or is suspected of favouring, one side. To be trusted and respected, he has to be seen to be impartial. The only side he can be allowed to show allegiance to is the health centre side; and it is the interests of the health centre that he has to promote and defend, not necessarily those of his supervisors. This does not mean that in any dispute between someone in the centre and an outsider, he must always align himself with the former against the latter. The interests of the health centre may not always coincide with the wishes of everyone who happens to be working in it. The health centre manager has to be concerned with the health centre as a whole, and he has to be able to appreciate everybody's point of view. If he feels that the health authority is itself damaging the health centre, or holding back its progress, he has to feel free to say so—however tactfully. Therefore, if authority over him is vested exclusively in the health authority, the responsible officers have to display a great deal of restraint and generosity if he is to be able to do his job effectively. Ideally, he should be answerable to both the health authority and a committee representing all those who work in the centre, and neither of these should have the power to fire him without the agreement of the other.

To repeat what has already been said, in order to play a full part in making the health centre a success, the health centre manager should be involved in the project as early as is practicable: certainly, well before the building comes into operation, and, ideally well before the design is finalised. If he is already involved with another health centre in the area, and will be taking on the new centre as an additional responsibility, it should be perfectly feasible to involve him from the very outset. Early involvement of the manager gives him an opportunity to gain the early acceptance and respect of the people who will be working in the new building; they cannot dismiss him as an outsider who only pokes his nose in when all the real work has been done. In the planning and design stages there is, in fact, a great deal of work for the health centre manager to do; having him there to ensure that it gets done can greatly increase the centre's chances of coming good.

The kind of tasks the health centre manager has to perform before and after the centre comes into operation are pretty much the same. At both times he has to ensure that communications channels are set up and maintained in good order, and that information flows freely. He has to ensure that everyone knows what is going on; that no-one is left in the dark, or feels that he is being left in the dark. Ignorance, or a *sense* of ignorance, about the health centre prevent a feeling of commitment to it, or involvement with it. He also has to ensure that all have an opportunity to air their grievances and express their opinions. It is his responsibility to prevent any group or individual being cowed into silence by dominant individuals. And he has to try to make sure that people with a grievance do not simply bottle up their grumbles instead of letting them out freely. Bottled up grumbles have a habit of eventually exploding with a big bang, and they can knock sizeable lumps off innocent by-standers who happen to be in the vicinity. Little annoyances, if dealt with as they come up, can leave a practice team's satisfaction with the health centre virtually unscathed. But if those little annoyances are neither expressed nor removed, they can eventually add up to an intolerable burden, and then—to everyone's surprise—doctors suddenly start talking about pulling out of the health centre altogether.

In any health centre, from time to time, there are inevitably going to be interpersonal disputes and dislikes. Most of the arguments will be trivial, but if allowed to get out of hand they can sour the whole atmosphere and involve everyone. The manager has to be able to stop them getting out of hand. He has to be a diplomatist, an arbitrator, and a conciliator. He has to be capable of getting people's confidence and trust, so that they are willing to talk to him and *want* to talk to him. He (or, if you like, she) has to be the sort of chap who people want to turn to when something goes wrong.

The health centre manager has to be quite a guy, or quite a gal. But where are such paragons to be found? At the moment, there is no obvious source of qualified recruits. All kinds of odd bods, with all kinds of backgrounds, seem to consider themselves ideally suited for the job—health authority officers among them. Health authority officers do have at least one virtue to recommend them: they know something (some less than others) about primary health care. This is important, because although the manager has to be able to handle interpersonal relationships, he also has to be a force for progress in the health centre. He has to be aware of the areas in which liaison might be improved, or new clinics or services profitably introduced. But the health authority officer has one big disadvantage: he is identified with one particular side. It is just about possible that he might be able to forget the loyalties and prejudices of his old job, and behave impartially in the new one; but even if he does succeed in this, no-one will believe that he has. A large part of those working in the health centre will forever watch him with suspicion and distrust.

The total outsider has the obverse advantages and disadvantages. He is unlikely to be accused of bias towards one side but, being a neophyte, his ignorance greatly limits his value. He cannot become of real value until he has learned a great deal, and if he is a slow learner he is likely to be promoted out of the health centre before he can do any good at all. However experienced he might be at handling people, he cannot begin to understand them until he appreciates the way the folk with whom he has to deal think, the way the world looks from their separate points of view, and their stereotypes of each other. The principles of human relationship may be the same in a health centre, or a factory, or an army barracks, but the detail differences are important too. The manager cannot get anywhere until he understands what doctors think of bureaucrats, and what social workers think of GPs. He is unlikely to get very far by recalling how he dealt with a strike of warpers and benders at his last place of work, or how he ended that unfortunate business at RAF Cranberry. Unless he knows the aspirations and dislikes, the values and fears, of all who work in the health centre, he is not going to appreciate that solutions which seem the most efficient on the face of it are certain to turn out the very opposite in practice. The old idea of doctors sharing consulting rooms is a good example. He has to learn what is *desirable* in the delivery of primary health care, but also has to learn what is *feasible.* If he tries to get things done too quickly he may be heading for disaster, particularly as he is open to the charge of being a newcomer and therefore not knowing what he is talking about.

A good health centre manager treads carefully to begin with, but, as in most situations, the sensible course can be pursued too far until it does not make sense any more.

One unfortunate gentleman made this error. When he was interviewed for the post of health centre manager, his self-confidence seemed quite adequate, but once the health centre opened this proved to be far from true. He was terrified of making a mistake, and had a kind of preoccupation with his own ignorance. He took the view that he could only begin to do his job when he was fully acquainted with everyone in the centre, everyone outside who was connected with it, and the details of their activities. He felt that if he said anything before he had this information, he would be laughed down and condemned forever. He decided that he needed time.

He refrained from doing anything until he was completely ready. He did not sort out a single problem or pour oil on any troubled waters, although the early months of the health centre offered plenty of opportunities for him to do so. Other people—a couple of enthusiastic GPs in particular—had to try to do his job instead. And this annoyed them more than a little, particularly since they were the ones who had argued the case for a health centre manager when many had considered the position to be entirely unnecessary. They considered that he had let them down—had actually made fools of them.

At the end of two years, he decided that he was ready to start earning his salary. He had lots of ideas, and thought that he knew how to get them implemented. But as he was deciding this, a committee sat to review the need for a health centre manager. They, not surprisingly, came to the conclusion that no such need had been demonstrated. The health centre had survived the relatively turbulent early days without his active help, and could look forward now to a reasonably problem-free future. So it seemed, anyway. As the manager was offered an even better-paid job elsewhere in the administration, he certainly did not argue. He did not suffer as a result of his mistake—but the health centre did.

The health centre manager has to learn, but he has to learn quickly, because he is most necessary in the months of preparation leading up to the opening of the centre, and in its first few years of life.

Worker Control

A health centre needs a full-time individual concerned with its integration and progress. But health centre management is not just a job for the health centre manager. If the centre is to be a success, everyone who works in it has to be involved in the management of its day-to-day operation and its development. The principal role of the health centre manager is to help and encourage them to do this. He is not there to try to play dictator.

There are many people working in, or otherwise connected with, health centres who argue that there is no need for any kind of management committee, let alone for a full-time manager. In their own centre, they insist, there is no need to get together to solve problems because there are no problems; there is no need for discussion, because there is nothing to discuss. But this is never true. What they take to be the truth is strictly illusion.

In any social situation as complex as a health centre, there are bound to be problems at least part of the time. If there is no opportunity to mention them, and get them dealt with, they will continue beneath the surface, unsuspected by any except those whom they directly affect. All the time they continue, they will impede the work of those whom they do affect, and in the bosoms of the latter they will cause an accumulation of annoyance. One day, this accumulation may become too great, and something dramatic will happen. If and when it does, great will be the surprise. But until then, all those destined to be surprised will be insisting that there is no need for the health centre to have a management committee, because nobody would have anything to say.

This health centre had been in operation for six months without a management committee or anything approaching it. For some reason, however, it was decided to hold a meeting now. No-one seemed to know where the idea had come from, and no-one admitted to considering such a meeting to be necessary. The common view was that there were no problems worth discussing, and everyone wondered what they would manage to talk about when they did have their meeting.

In the event, most of the eleven doctors in the centre attended, and the receptionists were asked to provide a delegate. The treatment room nurse was also invited, and one of the health visitors invited herself. The meeting began at 7p.m. and did not finish until after eleven.

All declared themselves to be amazed at the number of matters that had come to light during that time: the number of problems that had, in fact, been raised; and the number that had been sorted out.

The meeting had not been entirely amicable. Some unsuspected grievances had emerged, and given rise to hostility. But none of the arguments lasted for long, and it was agreed that the meeting had been a useful safety valve if nothing else. However, it did achieve much more. The use of the treatment room was re-organised; a source of discontent in the reception area was removed; communications with health authority officers concerned with the centre were improved; two new clinics were introduced; and an agreement to meet again regularly was made.

A management committee is often considered unnecessary for the surprising reason that nothing happens in the health centre anyway. Things go on as they have always done, and as a committee has not been required in the past, there would be no purpose in having one in the future. It *is* surprising because the fact that nothing happens in the centre is a good reason for *having* a management committee, not doing without one: unless, of course, everybody in the centre is happy that things should stay as they are, and have no wish for change. But often the lack of progress and development, the failure of the centre to produce any worthwhile innovation in ways of working, is a disappointment to many who moved into the centre in a spirit of optimism. They do not applaud the apparent permanence of the status quo, they merely take it for granted, just as they once took it for granted that the health centre would automatically make things different. Neither progress nor stagnation are inevitable, and everything depends on how the people concerned go about things. If they get together with the deliberate intention of discussing their health centre and how they can make better use of it, they will find the effort worthwhile. If they cannot be bothered to do this, they have only themselves to blame if the centre fails to be the paradise they had expected it to be.

There is even a case for a management committee in a health centre whose personnel are happy with the way things are, and have no unfulfilled ambitions for change. The manager who nags and cajoles until a committee is set up may find that he has wasted his time, but he may not. People are often satisfied with their present way of doing things because they are unaware of the alternative possibilities. Once they start talking to each other, hearing each other's ideas, and learning from each other, they may well find that there is scope for improvement. With the right kind of encouragement sleepy traditionalists can, and sometimes do, become progressives of almost embarrassing ardour.

All who work in a health centre are going to be more concerned with making the most of the opportunities it provides the more they identify with the health centre as a whole, and the less they consider themselves to constitute entirely independent units totally unrelated to, and unconcerned about, each other. Once they have recognised themselves to be all in the same boat, and sharing common interests, they may start to think about ways in which they can work more effectively together and the centre can be used to provide a better service for their patients. Apart from practical achievements which the management committee might make in these directions, it has value simply by virtue of its existence in that it helps to create and maintain a sense of solidarity. Once the committee has been set up, therefore, it tends to maintain its own impetus. Because they regularly meet with each other, health centre personnel consider themselves as part of the health centre, not just members of diverse professions or teams, and so they take an interest in the place as a whole, instead of only concerning themselves with their own particular affairs. At least, that is how it should work out.

Committee meetings will not always be harmonious, and

contact does not always lead to mutual affection. Individuals who could tolerate each other when they did not have to confront each other face to face might become frankly hostile when forced to meet across the committee table. And there is inevitably going to be argument, even among comparative friends. In most debates, disagreement usually crops up at least as often as agreement. But sensible and intelligent adults can tolerate this without losing their liking and respect for each other, and a decent health centre manager should be able to calm the situation down if it looks like getting out of hand. People who cannot be on the same committee without engaging in bitter acrimony would hopefully not be in the same health centre, having realised this fact when attending planning meetings, and consequently changing their plans before it was too late.

If the management committee is to be truly integrative, if it is to encourage all who work in the centre to *identify with* the centre and to recognise that they are all responsible for its fate, then it has to *represent* all. It should not be a selective body made up of members of only one profession, and from which everyone else is excluded. It is common practice when considering who should be on such a committee to assume that GPs and representatives of the health authority have a *right* to membership, and then perhaps to consider who else might be reasonably included without causing too much inconvenience to the 'proper' members. Insofar as it reflects the realities of power, this approach may make a kind of sense, but it is entirely the wrong way to go about the matter if the intention is to aim at a *successful* health centre, and not to be merely pragmatic. Success for a health centre depends on the efforts and inclinations of everyone connected with it, and not a single person should feel that he (she) is being left out in the cold. So, as far as the management committee is concerned, it is necessary to start with the assumption that *everyone* has a right to membership.

In larger centres particularly, there will be practical reasons why every single individual cannot sit at the same table and constitute the committee. This problem was discussed earlier* in the context of health centre planning. The solutions suggested

---

* Chapter 3.

there apply here, and there is no need to repeat them, but this at least should be re-stated: if some people are only allowed their say at management committee meetings in a vicarious fashion, those who represent them have to be effective representatives and truly representative. They have to be elected, not self-selected, and they have to ensure that their respective elector-tates are kept informed of what is said at the meetings, as well as ensuring that they keep themselves informed of what their electorates want. The selection of people who will actually sit on the committee has to be properly and democratically organised; and a good system of communications between them and everyone else in the health centre is absolutely essential.

Democratic health centre government can only happen if those who already have power are prepared to share it with those who do not. The health authority and the GPs could maintain an oligarchy if they so wished. Conceivably, the health authority might even try to exclude the GPs. It might begin in a spirit of enlightened generosity, and change its mind after a time, trying to regain exclusive control of health centre affairs.

There is one large, and therefore costly, health centre which started its life with a very democratically organised system of management. The MoH whose baby this centre was, was anxious to see it thrive, and realised that it would only do so if he handed it over freely to the many people who would be working in it. He told them that it was their health centre, and they were responsible for it. Decisions as to its development were theirs to make, and he would not interfere. As a result, there was more than the usual amount of pride and interest in their health centre among the nurses, doctors, social workers, sec-retaries and others in the place. Slowly perhaps, but perceptibly, things began to happen. Doctors and social workers even arranged joint talks on topics of common interest. The provision of new services within the centre was discussed. At Christmas there was a pantomime. Then, one day, somebody reorganised the health service. The MoH was gone, and responsibility for the centre was allocated to a new administrator who did not care to share his power with the health centre's own man-agement committee. So he told its members frankly that they had no authority, and might as well leave everything to him, for he would decide everything anyway. The barriers went up. But not where they might have been expected to go. It was not a case of the entire health centre population standing firm against this upstart administrator. Far from it. They seemed to accept that this battle was lost, and retreated to the lines they knew they could defend. They retreated back into their own practices and professional groups. The man might be able to veto their proposal for some new clinic to be held in the centre, but he could not tell the doctors what to do as far as their own practices were concerned, nor could he interfere in the work of the nurses, or the health visitors, or social workers. In defending themselves against this new attack, they put up barriers between themselves, barriers which they had spent the last few years in bringing down. By challenging the management committee's authority, the administrator did grave damage to the sense of solidarity and shared purpose that had developed in this health centre. The damage may well prove to be irreparable.

Having a fully-representative management committee is not the only way of promoting integration, but it tends to be the sine qua non. The health centre which organised a pantomime as part of its Christmas festivities has been mentioned. Where the people working in the centre already take a keen interest in their common premises, and have a strong sense of shared involvement, they may well decide to indulge in some pretty sophisticated social activities. Where there is no representative management committee, and where a sense of mutual responsibility for the centre is lacking, social gatherings can still occur, but tend to be much more strained affairs. If people really do work and plan together, they may well want to occasionally play together—or something like it. If they do *not* work and plan together, social gatherings seem rather irrelevant and, when they occur, are tolerated more out of a sense of duty than anything else. Here the Christmas gathering usually proves to be an embarrassing affair, as individuals congregate strictly in practice or professional groups and reaffirm rather than weaken the lines that divide the health centre.

Where everyone in the health centre is already involved in its management, informal social functions can help to strengthen the sense of solidarity that already exists. They are not indispensable. If people do not want them, they can manage quite well without them. There are some who feel that working with others eight hours a day is quite enough, without spending leisure time with them too. But they can allow everybody to get

135

to know each other rather better than they can from simply working alongside each other. At least, they can allow them to discover a side of each other they had not suspected before. Discoveries of this kind can change people's opinions of each other, and forge new bonds where none had existed before. After all, if it had not been for the party they had to celebrate the first birthday of a certain Health Centre, most people might have gone on thinking that Miss Bone the senior nursing officer was a bitter and inhuman creature, totally unapproachable and without an ounce of feeling, whereas now they know that she is quite capable of letting her hair down when the occasion allows it. Yes, the health centre life can be fun. It can be a lot of fun, if everybody goes about things the right way.

CHAPTER EIGHT

And in Conclusion

Most health centres, at first glance, might seem healthy enough. The patients are seen, and dealt with in a fashion. It is only from time to time that you hear of things being markedly worse than they were before the centre was built; only from time to time that you hear of a practice team breaking up, or friends becoming enemies as a result of the move. But health centres are not supposed to be merely no worse than what went before. They are meant to represent, encourage, and facilitate progress, and by this criterion of their well-being most of them, in fact, are pretty sick. A fair number are, literally, dead on their feet.

Considering their cost, and the effort that goes into making them, health centres ought to provide the very best, the most up-to-date and the most innovative, of primary health care. They ought to be the undisputed vanguard, marking a path for others to follow. What goes on within their walls ought to be worthy of attention, worthy of emulation and replication, manifestly superior to anything ever achieved outside. But what goes on within the great majority of health centres is hardly different from what was to be found previously, in the separate GP surgeries and health authority clinics.

Perhaps, for the most part, they are an improvement as far as comfort is concerned. Perhaps they impress the patients. Perhaps these things matter. It still cannot be denied that health centres in general, in this country, are, fundamentally, failures. They have failed to achieve what they have all along been intended to achieve: the closer, more serious, more effective working together of the various individuals and services involved in the delivery of primary health care.

It has too often been taken for granted that simply putting as many people as possible under the one roof would inevitably lead to more contact and communication amongst them; that there would, as a result, be more appreciation of each other's skills and role, more frequent and more speedy referral of patients, better feedback of information, less unnecessary replication. It has too often been taken for granted that health centres are inevitably good for the patient because they not only provide a variety of people to work for him, they ensure that those people will work *together* for him. But few health centres, in practice, have displayed a great deal of togetherness, and it is more usual to find individuals operating in as much isolation as they did before the centre was built.

Although it is obviously desirable that all who work within a health centre should work in co-operation with each other, and make the most of each other's close proximity, it is *most* important that all should be well within the individual primary health care teams. Some patients can benefit from the GP (for example) having a satisfactory relationship with the chiropodist or speech therapist in the centre, but considerably more are dependent for their welfare upon satisfactory relationships inside the practice team.

Happily, the majority of doctors, receptionists, and attached health visitors, midwives and nurses are committed to their own practice teams, and anxious that they should not lose their identity in new health centre premises. If their team is not threatened, they are more likely to see the potential of the health centre, and to be willing to work more closely with everyone else with whom they share the building. But it they see the centre as a threat to the team, they will, as like as not, resent the presence of all non-members, and reinforce the boundaries between themselves and the rest. This is why the two goals of good primary health care teams and good teamwork across the health centre as a whole have a tendency to suffer the same fate: either they are both achieved or neither of them is.

Good things can only happen in health centres if people want them to happen and if they are prepared to put in the effort to make them happen. Health centres cannot exert an automatic effect; they cannot *determine* what will happen to relationships within their walls. But they can do a lot to influence what people themselves want, and they can do a lot to determine how much effort those people will have to expend in order to achieve what they want.

A health centre should encourage the lukewarm or indifferent to see the benefits of closer liaison with personnel whom they had previously been happy to largely ignore. Instead, it is more likely to discourage even the enthusiastic advocates of team-work. A health centre should make it easy for the team, to operate together as a team, and to communicate with everybody else in the centre. Instead, it is more likely to put obstacles in their way, and to make them feel that there are better things to spend their time and energy upon.

By the time that a health centre is opened, much should already have been done to try to ensure that those who move into it will want to do their best to put the centre to good use. In practice nothing of the kind will have been done, and a fair proportion of the incoming population will have no enthusiasm for the place at all, or will quickly become disappointed with it. It is important to realise that among GPs in particular (and this does not apply only to the more ancient members of the profession) hopes and fears attached to health centres in the past often colour present-day attitudes. Apprehension of loss of professional freedom and health authority takeover is still quite widespread. On the other hand, there are those who still preserve the idea that a health centre will provide technological hardware, and give the doctor higher status by allowing him to do something at least of what is now done in hospitals. If the health authority wants its health centres to be a success, it should do its best to demonstrate that it has no dishonourable intentions as far as the general practitioners are concerned, and it should demonstrate to those hoping for the wrong benefits precisely what the health centre can provide, and in what ways it can enhance the GPs' esteem.

A good way of achieving both these things is to involve the doctors along with everyone else concerned with the centre in the process of health centre planning. There are other advantages too in making the planning process completely democratic. It is not always easy to attain this, particularly where large numbers of people are involved, but it can be done by having representatives of each practice team and professional or occupational group involved at every planning meeting, by having proper election of representatives, and by ensuring adequate feedback of information to the represented. A health centre manager can take on much of the burden of organising this if he is brought on the scene at such an early date.

Administrators are apt to argue that the fewer people who are involved in the planning of a health centre the better: time is saved, and that means money is saved too. But often, keeping out all but a privileged few, turns out to be expensive. Even the most experienced architect needs to know just how the people who will be working in the health centre *propose* to work in it. If he produces his design without bothering to consult them in detail, he risks creating a building which will be a constant source of frustration to its incumbents, and which may have to be altered at considerable cost in the future. If it proves impossible to alter it, the frustrations it causes will result in everyone working less effectively than they might have done, and that represents an expense too. The health centre will not be providing the fullest possible value for the money spent on its construction.

Getting value for money out of the health centre involves getting *everyone* who works in it to want to make the most of it. They have to regard the health centre as something for which they are themselves responsible, and they have to be encouraged to think of ways in which they can realise the potential it offers. But they are much more likely to regard the place as *their* health centre, and much more likely to be concerned for its future, if they have themselves been encouraged to play a full and active part in its planning. If the health centre is simply provided for them, if they are landed with somebody else's ideas rather than allowed to express their own, they cannot be blamed for taking no pride in it and feeling no responsibility for it.

Much of the health centre's potential lies in its capacity to allow people with diverse skills and functions in primary health care to co-operate with each other and to learn from each other. To that end, no opportunity should be lost to bring everyone together and to establish some sense of unity. The first, and in many ways the best, opportunity to do this comes *before* the health centre is in operation, when the project is in the planning stage. Sitting together in committee meetings, talking and arguing about the health centre, gives people the chance to get to know each other, and to get to know what they each expect from their new premises. A further advantage is that if someone decides that he is not going to be able to get on with the rest, or that his own ideas about the health centre are incompatible with everybody else's, he can pull out before it becomes too difficult to do so.

Participation in the planning should not be restricted to those who have enough power and interest to demand a say. The success of the health centre requires that everyone be involved, even those who have no particular wish to be. The indifferent and the downright antagonistic have to be *encouraged* to take part, even if the meetings do inevitably become more difficult as a result. At least there will be a chance of winning them over to the health centre cause, and dispelling their suspicions. If they are simply left out in the cold, they are likely to become even less enthusiastic about the project.

The principal aim of the planning process, of course, is to come up with a decent design for the health centre: a design that will contribute to the attainment of both goals, the promotion of the primary health care team and the encouragement of overall teamwork. Because overall teamwork is only likely to develop if the individual practice teams feel secure, this really means designing for the primary health care team. But when you look at most health centre plans, you might be forgiven for thinking that the intention was to break up the team rather than to help it. Instead of all the members being put in the same part of the building, they are scattered all over the place and compelled to share rooms with people who do not belong to the team at all.

A practice is fortunate indeed if it has its own waiting and receptions areas. In all probability it will have to share space with every other practice in the centre, and possibly with the receptionists serving the various health authority services too. It is generally assumed that what is done with the receptionists does not matter to the primary health care team, but this assumption is gravely wrong. The receptionist is a key member of the team, and the area in which she works is a key area.

When the practice is in its own premises, the receptionist will be in a position to collect and relay messages from (and to) all the other members of the team. The doctor, the nurse, the midwife, and the health visitor will all call into the reception area from time to time, and occasionally will do so simultaneously. Consequently, the receptionist and her work-space constitute a point of contact for the team as a whole. But if she is forced to share space with all the other receptionists in the health centre, and if she is plonked down at some distance from the doctor, the nurse, the midwife and the health visitor, her contact with them will almost inevitably suffer, and so will her ability to serve as a centre of communications. Furthermore, the other team members may well be reluctant to come into the reception area because it is shared with other practices, and therefore lose a lot of opportunity for accidental contact with each other.

If the practice does not have its own reception and waiting areas its identity suffers in the eyes of the patient, and communications between patient and receptionist, and patient and GP, can suffer too. Because of her relative isolation, the receptionist may well feel less involved with the practice team, less committed to it, and less inclined to put herself out on its behalf. Physical dispersal, in general, does terrible things to team solidarity.

It is not only the receptionists who have a habit of being cut off from the rest of the primary health care team in health centres. The nurse, the health visitor and the midwife can find themselves stuck in isolated outposts as well. It is usual practice to make all the nurses in the centre share a single room, and the same applies to the health visitors and midwives. It makes a kind of sense to do this, particularly in economic terms. But it plays havoc with the primary health care team. It discourages contact—particularly *personal*, direct contact—and it reinforces feelings that there remain two, ultimately distinct sides—the GP side and the health authority side—precluding the possibility of a truly integrated team. The interests of the practice team require that all the health authority personnel attached to a practice should have, at least, a single room for them to share alongside the consulting rooms of the doctors with whom they work.

It would seem to go without saying that if the team is to be a team, and is to work as a team, then it should have somewhere to *meet* as a team. It might seem to go without saying, but it is rarely acknowledged in health centre design. The health centre common room is treated as indispensable, even though it is usually inadequately used, but no-one is apparently inclined to

142

let each practice team have its own meeting room. Yet to do so would be of great value to the team—and it could be said that *without* somewhere to meet together, the various members cannot really function as a team at all: they cannot properly co-ordinate their activities, they cannot make the fullest use of their joint skills. On top of this, instead of discouraging contact with other people in the centre, giving each practice team somewhere to meet in private would probably make them less resentful of non-members and more willing to develop wider contacts. They might well use the health centre common room more, instead of less. The objection of cost might be overcome by devising means of partitioning off the practice waiting area outside surgery hours, thereby avoiding the need for a separate room.

Decorations and furnishings can do their bit to preserve the identities of the separate practices in a health centre. There is no reason why every part of the building should be painted the same colour, or why every room should look the same. A patchwork quilt effect would be visually much more entertaining. And if a doctor wants to bring in with him some relic from his old surgery (apart from the receptionists) why not let him, as long as he does not end up with his consulting room stacked to the ceiling like an auctioneer's showroom.

Physical surroundings can make a lot of difference, but walls are not the only constraints upon what people in health centres can get up to. Very few are free agents. Most come under the authority of others so they cannot always do just what they want to do. They cannot develop their working relationships with each other entirely according to their own inclination. Senior nursing officers and people of similar kind are by no means always a brake on progress towards teamwork, but sometimes they are, and sometimes they are believed to be. Disputes between GPs and those responsible for the nurse, health visitor or midwife attached to their practice are not as rare as they ought to be—not by a long way. Often the fault is on the GP's side, often it is on both sides, and more often than not the fault lies in a lack of thought rather than in fundamental disagreement or personal antipathy.

If the people directly concerned with the delivery of primary health care are to work well together, all those with authority over them have to work well together too. They have to communicate freely with each other, be open with each other, and be willing to discuss ways in which the practice team and overall health centre teamwork can be developed. Insofar as their subordinates are supposed to be part of a broader set-up in the health centre, not simply being concerned with their own particular role and expertise, they themselves have to think beyond the confines of their own immediate area of responsibility, and be prepared to recognise the rights of others to comment on things which do come within that area. Teamwork on the ground depends on teamwork at the higher levels.

Where the doctor's receptionists are taken on to the pay-roll of the health authority when the health centre is opened, it is equally important that whoever is put in charge of them should work very closely with the GPs and other team members. This is particularly so when a new receptionist has to be appointed. Reception and secretarial staff are vital members of the primary health care team, and if the doctors no longer employ them it is essential that they should still be allowed to work with their original practices. The advantages of rotating receptionists around all the practices are trivial compared to the damage that is thereby done to the individual teams themselves. Ideally, of course, the GPs should hang onto their own ladies, and if they do not want to be bothered with the associated administration, employ a practice manager or some such person to do it for them.

Even if the GPs do continue to employ their own receptionists, when the time comes to hire a new one they should give consideration to how well the recruit will fit in with everyone else in the health centre. It is not enough that she should be able to get on with members of her own team. This is particularly true where she has to share a reception area with other practices, because if she is involved in constant dispute her own work will suffer. But even where each practice has its own reception and waiting areas, care should be taken not to bring in anyone who will rock the health centre boat. This is in everybody's interest—including that of the doctors who do the hiring. And, naturally, similar thought should be given to anyone else who might be brought into the health centre once it has got under way: nurses, health visitors, or doctors. It makes no sense at all to disrupt a health centre which has settled down nicely by introducing someone who is bound to cause trouble.

There is an equally strong case for vetting everyone who proposes to come into the health centre at the outset. Some people are so incompatible that they will never be able to co-exist peacefully under the same roof, and allowing them into the health centre is a good way of ensuring the centre's failure. It is by no means always easy to spot those who will violently disagree, because even friends can find that too much physical proximity turns them against each other, but involving everyone in the planning process and allowing them to discuss the proposed health centre in detail together, can provide an opportunity for major disagreements to be discovered before it is too late. For the sake of the health centre, and for the sake of the individuals themselves, it may be best for some people to be actively discouraged from moving into the centre. Perhaps some people should be actively discouraged from moving into any health centre.

The health centre will only be a success if all those who work in it, and all those who exercise authority over them, want it to be a success. But wanting is not enough in itself. Effort has to be made: properly directed effort. And somebody has to be responsible for co-ordinating it. Maybe somebody who already has a job to do in the centre will take on this responsibility, for whatever reason, but it really requires a full-timer. It needs a health centre manager. Maybe one such individual could be concerned with two or three health centres if they are small enough, but in the case of larger centres a one-to-one ratio is essential. The manager has such a lot to do: he has to be concerned with ensuring that all goes smoothly for the practice teams in the centre, and he has to try to encourage improved working relationships across the health centre as a whole. He has a responsibility for ensuring that the fullest use is made of the centre, that its potential is realised to the greatest possible extent. He has a lot of responsibility, but he probably has no power at all: no authority over anyone else in the building. So he has to create his own authority by gaining the respect of others. If he cannot gain their respect, he might as well not be employed, because he will be incapable of exerting any effect—at least, any effect for the good. So the health centre manager has to be chosen very, very carefully. It is a long way from being the sort of job that anyone can tackle with success.

A health centre manager is necessary, but he (or she) is only there to help everyone else in the health centre to manage it for themselves. By one means or another, all who work in the place should be encouraged to take a hand in deciding how it should be operated, and how the services that it provides might be developed in the future. There has to be a proper, democratic, health centre management committee, even if at first there does not appear to be any need for it, even if it seems that nobody will have anything to say. Setting up such a committee is very often what is necessary to get people thinking and talking about their health centre, and considering how they can make the best possible use of it.

There will only be development of the primary health care team, there will only be decent teamwork encompassing the centre as a whole, there will only be improvement and extension of health centre services for the benefit of the patient, if all those who actually work in the building consider this to be *their* health centre, and regard themselves as being responsible for its welfare. If the health authority wants its centres to be a success, wants them to provide maximum value for money, it has to avoid giving the impression that it is firmly in charge, and that what the individual nurse or receptionist or GP has to say does not matter.

'Making sick health centres better' has two meanings. Firstly, it means making better those health centres which are already in operation, but which are not looking too rosy. If they are considered honestly, many of the health centres extant in this country fall into this category. Hopefully, much of what has been said in the preceding pages will provide some indications as to therapy. No cure is guaranteed, of course, because some cases may well be too far gone already, or may even suffer from maladies that have not been considered here. But, with a bit of luck, there will be some improvement in the condition.

The second meaning of the phrase refers to making better health centres from the start, and obviously there is much more chance of success if things can be tackled properly from the first stage of the project. As has been said, the way the planning process is handled can have a lot to do with how well or otherwise the health centre fares when it is actually built.

This book has dealt pretty well exclusively with health authority-built centres, for the simple reason that most health centres are of this type. But most of what has been said is relevant to GP-owned centres too. It is just that the doctors themselves have to take responsibility for doing much that has been urged upon health authority administrators. They have to ensure that planning and management are properly handled, that a decent design is worked out, and that disruptive characters are kept out of the centre. They still have to work closely with senior nursing officers, senior social workers, etc., if they are to make best use of the premises they have invested so much capital in. Merely owning your own building does not guarantee success or automatically eliminate all possible problems. A consortium of GPs can still fall out amongst themselves if the autonomy and identity of their separate practices is not safeguarded in the centre, or if they fundamentally disagree on ways in which the centre might be developed.

It would be pleasing to conclude by saying that the greatest hope for the future lies in the new generation of people who are now going through training in the various branches of primary health care. It would be comforting to think that they are, at this very moment, being educated to work together and to realise the potential of health centres. But, sadly, there is not as much sign of this as there really ought to be. On the contrary, there seems to be a pre-occupation with turning out new doctors, or nurses, or anything else one cares to name, who think precisely like their seniors. Indeed, and this is the biggest tragedy, the neophytes themselves seem anxious to imitate their older fellow-professionals in order to gain their acceptance. Consequently, young people are still coming into health centres who are sometimes no more inclined to make proper use of them than are the most reactionary of those already *in situ*. Something will have to be done about it.

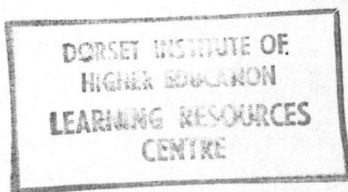

147